ADDICTED
TO THE SUN

BOOK OF MIRACLES

CAPTAIN LEO WALTON

NEWMAN SPRINGS PUBLISHING
320 Broad Street
Red Bank, NJ 07701

First originally published by Newman Springs Publishing 2020

ISBN 978-1-64801-813-8 (Paperback)
ISBN 978-1-64801-814-5 (Digital)

Printed in the United States of America

To my guru, Hira Ratan Manek, who by his extraordinary efforts on researching ancient sungazing methods and creating a safe effective system for the betterment of humankind, without his influence and encouragements, I would not be as healthy and illuminated as today. In our last communication, when I was detailing my efforts to teach his methods—the HRM protocol, Hira said, "Please spread this message to humanity to the maximum extent possible with my best wishes."

This is my response: "Hira, I'm doing my best."

Contents

Introduction

A brief bio about me and how I became interested in sungazing.

I am Captain Leo Walton, and my last career was as a successful consultant, a self-employed marine forensics investigator for fifteen years representing nineteen different insurance companies. I performed over two thousand five hundred investigations and was contracted to work for periods of time on seven different hurricane catastrophe teams. My specialties were broad in scope; I performed mechanical failure analysis, oil spill containments, recovery of sunken vessels, lightning investigations, fire investigations, injury and wrongful death investigations, accident investigations, and was a court room expert witness.

My career was cut short when I experienced an accident aboard my own vessel while working on the electrical shore power system.

Since that time following my recovery, I utilized my skills as an independent researcher, and as a part of my research, I have been doing aggressive hands on experimentation and investigations on subtle energies.

Over the past decade, my focus and intentions of my research are a direct result of symptoms related to an electric shock. The two hundred twenty-volt AC, fifty-amperage electricity arced from an electrical panel, entering my left hand, and raced through the left hemisphere and frontal lobes of my brain, causing severe traumatic brain injury, damaging both my pituitary and pineal glands to the point of dysfunction.

It took a year for me to regain the ability to read. I could recognize and read the words individually, but I couldn't put together the meaning of the statement; the words were just another foreign language I couldn't interpret.

The electric shock evoked a sudden kundalini awakening and NDE.

For many months following my "grand Illumination," I like to call it. I had lost the sense of touch of my body. I couldn't feel the warmth of the sun on my face, I couldn't feel the wind blowing through my hair, and I was numb inside as a human being as well.

One thing that wasn't absent was pain. The myelin coating which covers our nerves like plastic insulation on wiring was melted off those neural pathways which were used as conduit of the AC current due to the intense heat of the electrical arc, which required 2600 degrees Fahrenheit to melt the stainless-steel bracelet loose from my wrist.

However, just as quickly that my senses left me, when they returned, it was with an equally instant flash that was profound and acute.

The brief excitement and short-lived celebration of being able to feel my own flesh again diminished soon afterwards, turning to horror as my body physically reacted with involuntary twisting and contorting and agony consumed me. The reactions I experienced were violent as I was attacked by the relentless resonance frequency vibrations of the reciprocating compressor motor when my refrigerator cycled on. The alien and tormenting physical sensations I suffered at that moment were debilitating, and I began an unchartered adventure which I did not volunteer or agree to.

Most of the education I have gained since has evolved from over a decades research, with hands-on experimentation with ancient and modern methods such as sungazing, breatharianism, prescription drugs, radioniçs, blood electrification, yoga, reiki, deep meditation states, brainwave entrainment, astral travel, visiting over forty medical doctors, psychologists, and psychiatrists. Add to that list my own lengthy encounters of unnatural experiences including paranormal, which were fueled by a super intuitive ability to source information.

For the longest time, the only general medical response I received from those I sought help from was that I was a miracle man, and nobody honestly knew what to do with me. I was supposed to be dead.

Fast-forward to present.

From the moment I was electrocuted and active today, my life has been 100 percent centered around energy, frequency, and vibration. With little information available at the time from western medicine, I sourced alternative methods to help me regain some form of stability in my life. I trained in yoga for the physical therapeutic benefits and immersed myself into the eastern philosophies, becoming a trained yogi and using the abundance of ancient skills and wisdom I discovered as a source of invaluable information. This provided me with much healing I so desperately needed at the time. Even with the devotion and continued improvements I gained, my bio-energies became more manageable, but they were still not under my command. It seemed that the rogue energies had a mind of their own, and I was just a passenger along for the ride. It was not until I began to train in the Japanese healing art known as reiki, becoming a reiki master, that I finally gained a level of confidence and skill manipulating my own bio-energy fields I was comfortable with.

I learned over time that I could feel not only industrial energy fields but also natural earth and cosmic energy streams as well. I developed the ability to close my eyes and slowly turn in a circle and identify all eight directions of the earth's electromagnetic fields just as accurately as a ship's magnetic compass. I have learned that because of this ability to feel electromagnetic streams that I am considered a magneto receiver or a geomancer.

Another interesting ability I gained is when the ships come into the harbor from the Atlantic Ocean near where I live—as they enter the harbor when it is foggy, and they sound their very loud and deep tuned fog horns, I learned during these instances that I could feel the sound before I could hear it, with such accuracy that I can tell another person when the horn will sound. Because of this relationship, I have become convinced and developed a theory that sound vibrations contain light and, therefore, is faster than light.

I later learned I could feel the sun's vibrational frequencies prior to sunrise and tell another individual the minute the sun has risen without being able to see it.

I learned I was sensitive to certain microwave antenna systems, being able to feel them and some being capable of hearing them when they were activated.

I have become pre-cognitive, I have visions, and I have gained free access to any and all information I have sourced at the appropriate moment to confirm what I already have known.

With that said, with my childlike curiosity and tenacious desire to learn, I found myself with thirteen manuscripts each in different phases of production, including hundreds of original drawings I sketched from the visuals I received. Currently my intentions are focused on production and the completion of these projects for publication, this manuscript being the first. From my earliest thoughts on writing and publication, my desires have been to offer a thoroughly researched, well-thought-out, well-presented, coherently described, and well-written series, which now includes multiple volumes.

Thousands of hours have been spent researching and drawing. I have produced thousands of journal pages with new perspectives on an eclectic range of topics, including the intent and purpose including systems operations of the Giza Pyramids, the termination of the Ice Age theories, on human cranial deformations, the Nazca Lines, and earth energy grid systems.

This first volume, Addicted to the Sun, will begin with a man's journey of examining energy from an entirely new perspective, and each successive volume will contribute to an overall the understanding of our cosmic and earthly fields related to quantum entanglement.

Once my nervous system had become accustomed and comfortable with the energies of my own bio-energy network and those of my environment, I was then afforded the luxury to examine other energy sources from a new perspective. I had no choice in the matter; my entire outlook on life in general was forced to change or die.

During my tenacious seeking, I learned of sungazing from the ancient Hindus, and when I had progressed to doing historical Egyptian research, I discovered additional information in the ancient symbols that led me to recognizing yet another culture that used sungazing as a tool and the different methods they had devised.

I became very interested and gave the topic a lot of attention. I was continually amazed at the healing benefits it promised by simply staring at the sun naked-eyed for a forty-four-minute duration. While extreme and farfetched, going against everything I had been taught, it sounded only short of a miracle to me.

Little did I realize at that time then, but my desperation was about to encourage me to become a very serious bio-hacker, allowing myself to be my own guinea pig. I like to laugh and say I became both Dr. Frankenstein and his creation, the monster.

In my pursuits, I left no stone unturned, experimenting with both ancient and modern methods to regain excellent health and to incorporate the methods to create a new identity for myself, which was lost due to my severe traumatic brain injuries.

General information

When it comes to our heart, a study done at Tulane University says sunlight lowers blood pressure. Those with normal blood pressure had a slight lowering, which lasted one or two days after exposure to sunlight. Those with high blood pressure had a great reduction of their blood pressure, and the effects lasted longer—five to six days. Sunlight lowers blood sugar and is most dramatic in people that are diabetics. It decreases the resting heart rate, increases cardiac output, increases cardiac stamina, and increases the storage of glycogen in the liver.

Sunlight is responsible for an increase in general energy, endurance, and muscular strength of the entire body. Ultraviolet light increases the bodies reaction to infections by producing increased production of lymphocytes and neutrophils, which are the basic chemical components of the immune system.

Go slow when it comes to sun exposure. Allow your eyes and your skin to adapt, avoiding burning. However, it is still a good idea to avoid prolonged sun exposure during the hours of 10:00 a.m. to 2:00 p.m. because of harmful radiation. Be smart, be in-tuned to your body, and listen to what it's telling you.

In regard to sun tanning products, they are more harm than good. The chemical compounds used to formulate the creams and oils are absorbed directly into the body, causing greater harm then the sun ever could.

The entire "protect your skin with sunblock" is being debunked daily.

The heart's efficiency improves, increasing blood flow volumes up to 29 percent when exposed to sunlight. This lasts again five to six days after exposure. Dramatic drops in serum cholesterol and triglyceride levels are not uncommon. Sunlight increases the oxygen carrying capacity of the blood.

The extra oxygen improves as a cleansing agent and removes dangerous particles from the blood system and encourages the body's immune system to function more efficiently. Cholesterol is actually destroyed by sunlight. As the cholesterol in the skin changes as a result to sunlight, it increases the amount of vitamin D storage in the body.

A Russian experiment proved that if the human skin is not exposed to solar radiation by direct or scattered means for long periods of time, disturbances of the physiological equilibrium of the human system will occur, the results being functional disorders of the nervous system, vitamin D deficiency, and a weakening of the bodies' defenses and an aggravation to chronic disease.

Concerning our eyes, when full spectrum of electromagnetic potential enters the eye, the optic facility works more productively. Light enters the eye to the optic nerve, which then stimulates the pineal gland which controls melatonin production. Our circadian rhythm keeps us in tune with the earth's natural cycles.

The wearing of sunglasses has recently been proven to be detrimental to one's over all wellbeing. Wearing sunglasses is like eating processed food; it alters the balance of nature's intentions.

They can actually cause mal-illumination, almost the same as malnutrition. Our eyes are designed to bring in light for nourishment for the nervous system and the cells. If we filter out the natural light, full-spectrum light, we are processing a limited spectrum of light which is the same as a fast food or processed food diet. So wearing of sunglasses is bad for your eyes and overall health. It may take some time for your eyes to adjust to the sunlight if you haven't allowed them to see the sun in a while.

(Note: This is exactly where I was. I wore sunglasses even at night. I did not have any eyewear that were not prescription sunglasses. Following my "grand illumination," my eyes were sensitive to all light—natural and man-made—plus add my cataracts from the increased protein production on my eye lenses from the electricity running through them when I was injured.)

The retina of human eye contains light sensitive cells—they are rods and cones. The rods are sensitive only to the intensity of the light, and the cones are only sensitive to color.

When it comes to our skin, doctors once again are re-evaluating and changing their thoughts when it comes to the sun and skin cancer. They have discovered it is more what is inside the human body that causes skin cancer than the exposure to the sun. With our unrefined western diets, various toxins in our system and even our unexpressed emotions contribute more to our aging process and to the development of cancer much more than the sun. Excessive sunlight can accelerate skin cancer if you already have it, but it is not the root cause.

The function of every cell in our body is controlled by electrical signals sent through our nervous system. Our nerves are an elaborate system of tiny waterways that carry electrically charged chemicals to every part of our body.

If the nerve pathways become dehydrated or contaminated, vital signs become distorted. These distorted signals may lead to degenerative diseases and neurological illnesses such as ADD and chronic fatigue syndrome, anxiety, depression, or Alzheimer's disease.

Significations pertaining to medical astrology

The sun has a bilious (pita) temperament. Its strength or weakness reflects the state of general health of an individual. It rules over the heart, stomach, bones, and right eye. The medical conditions that the sun rules over include, headache, baldness, hyperirritability, fevers, and pains, burns, diseases arising from inflammation of bile (like certain diseases of the liver and gallbladder), heart troubles, eye disease, stomach ailments, bone disorders, certain skin problems, injuries from falls, weapons and poisoning, disturbances of the blood circulation, epilepsy, leprosy, and fear of quadrupeds, thieves, and serpents.

It dries up moisture, killing harmful bacteria, and it keeps the environment clean. Solar rays are beneficial for those with a deficiency of vitamin D or from jaundice.

The sun is our nearest star in space with all the planets revolving around it. It is the source of all our natural light and heat of the earth. It provides the centripetal force to balance the centrifugal force generated by the planets going around it.

Sunbathing actually can increase the lungs' ability to absorb more oxygen as well as increase the bloods capacity to carry and deliver the oxygen.

Cancer and illness such as chronic fatigue syndrome thrive on the lack of sunlight.

Cells are bipolar like a battery—negative and positive.

Everything is a form of light, even matter, which is condensed light.

The human body is a photobiotic machine. It depends entirely on being able to absorb energy from different sources—electromagnetic, etheric, and electrochemical. Our health depends on it.

The color spectrum of light has a major influence on us as human creatures. The color red, for example, when using for long periods, can cause violent, fertile, aggressive behaviors. It can stimulate physical activity in an object and cause an increase in the fruition of plants, causing increased seed production.

The colors blue or green at the other end of the color spectrum can induce relaxation and sleep.

When a person is dying, the skin develops an ashen color just before death. As those in the east refer, "no color, no life."

Contact with these regions of lack of color on the dying will find the areas very cold and lacking warmth.

Practices such as yoga, sun-do, gigu, and pranic breathing all incorporate abdominal breathing to cleanse and invigorate the body with more energy.

The raw volume of prana or qi being emitted from the sun is beyond our comprehension.

Sunlight is responsible for an increase in general energy, endurance, and muscular strength of the entire body. When the sunlight penetrates the skin, it stimulates the entire molecular structure of the body. Ultraviolet light increases the body's reaction to infections by producing increased production of lymphocytes and neutrophils, which are the basic chemical components of the immune system.

Believe it or not, one of the most powerful medicines is drinking sun-drenched water (sun water or solar water). Letting a clear glass container set in the sun for between five to eight hours in direct sunlight gives the water a vibrational charge of the sun's energy.

They claim drinking a couple liters of this sun-energized water in the late afternoon on an empty stomach could help maintain remarkable health.

Ingesting this water may also bring the body's energy systems into balance.

Like sungazing, this is a form of medicine that is totally free.

A number of Eastern Indian medicines are prescribed to drink sun-drenched water. The use of colored bottles are also used to change the vibrational frequency of the water, to tailor it more for the individuals' health issues.

HRM recommends using different colored bottles with impressive results.

(Note: I experimented with different colored bottles for a while with my "rainbow water," but by the time I was at this research stage, I didn't suffer from any ailments I needed special attention on, so I tried them all to see if I could feel the difference if frequencies. At that time, I have to be honest and say I could not tell any significant frequency differences between the colors I tried in comparison to clear, but again, I would not claim it was the perfect methods I used.

This experiment should be repeated again, with isolating one color for a time period because the frequencies are subtle and will be slow in their reaction time.)

Thank you for letting me be your guide and taking the time to take this journey with me.

Chapter 1

Coronavirus: Death by Sunlight

The Research

I became very excited on April 28, 2020, when I received from the publisher their edit of my first manuscript for publication entitled, *Addicted to the Sun: Book of Miracles*, for my review.

Just the month before, the entire United States populace had been placed into a mandated martial law lockdown, making us prisoners inside our own homes because of the global pandemic known as the coronavirus or COVID-19.

On January 29, 2020, President Donald Trump established the White House Coronavirus Task Force, and a scientific research began by Homeland Security on studying the environments the COVID-19 thrived and what was the best environment to destroy it, along with other assorted methods including chemicals. Testing was performed at the US Army's high-level biosecurity laboratory at Fort Detrick, Maryland.

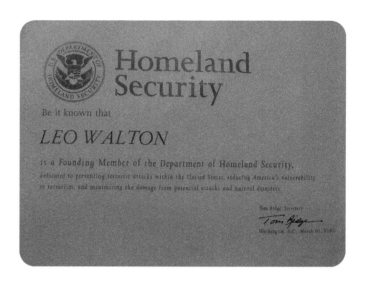

Only a few days earlier in the week, before I received the publisher's edit, William N. Bryan, the acting undersecretary for science and technology at the Homeland Security department, detailed recent lab studies carried out by the agency at the laboratory. Having been a founding member of Homeland Security, I was accustomed to watch these White House telecast at the time; and on that day, I viewed them on the official government White House website. I was particularly interested in the findings presented by the laboratory experiments performed by the scientist of Homeland Security.

At this same time frame, my fiancé, Heidi Grant (who provided the great photographs of sunrise from inside the Stonehenge at winter solstice on December 22, 2019, for the cover art of this book), who resides in London, was placed on quarantine lockdown by the UK government medical staff for fourteen days because she had become ill. Their decision obviously based on suspicions she had the coronavirus they determined from her conversation detailing the virus symptoms, which were numerous. They would not schedule her an appointment to see her physician at that time. I was greatly concerned for Heidi; she was bedridden and seriously ill for days by the time she contacted them for advice and help. I was already feeling guilty and responsible for her being sick because we suspected I may have had the coronavirus myself and infected her when she visited me in the US; I'll elaborate more on this scenario later.

One night, days following her contact with the medical services people, Heidi called me in a panic, struggling to breathe. Immediately, I recognized her behavior, having served two communities as a professional EMT trained firefighter, I know medical emergency rescue procedures, and I had determined my Heidi was in a state of hyperventilation. Because of my training and years of experience, I was luckily able to coach her on how to gain control of her breath.

In a few minutes, she had calmed and was able, even under stress, to communicate in her situation. I learned from her panicked lips some very frightening and concerning experiences she had suffered when she contacted the same emergency call number to get medical help because she couldn't breathe. The London operator told her that there were no emergency medical services available to her at the moment, and she could wait on hold on the line for the next twenty minutes or so to see if they would answer the call. The operator then instructed her to just continue with her quarantine for another seven days and then placed her on hold. Within five minutes, the phone call terminated, and Heidi was disconnected, cutting her off.

I must say I was experiencing a different kind of stress being in America under martial law and not being able to do anything to help the woman I loved and cared about so dearly. It was a helplessness in a way that was so powerful I had never experienced before. I was accustomed to provide excellent professional emergency care, and to witness firsthand another system pretty much to say, "No, we can't help. Just stay isolated at home for another week," and then cut her off is an absolute absurdity.

Let's say, I was real interested in what Homeland Security and Bryan had to say. The results were briefed to the press and on live television via slides largely matching other laboratory studies and the suspicions of some researchers by showing that the novel coronavirus, like many other viruses, does not survive as long on certain surfaces in the air are exposed to high amounts of ultraviolet light and warm and humid conditions.

The laboratory results show that increases in temperature, humidity, and sunlight—all can speed up how fast the virus is destroyed using half-life references to measure the death rate of the virus on different surfaces. For example, a slide presentation by Bryan revealed this finding applied to the virus in contact with nonporous surfaces such as door handles. Adding in the sunlight, the virus's half-life decreases from six hours to two minutes at a temperature from 70 to 75 degrees and humidity of 80 percent.

"That's how much of an impact UV rays has on the virus," Bryan said.

The laboratory experiment also tested how the virus decays when exposed to various elements while suspended in the air. When the airborne virus at temperatures between 70 to 75 degrees is exposed to sunlight, its half-life decreases from around sixty minutes before exposure to 1.5 minutes after.

Bryan summarized, "Within the conditions we've tested to date, the virus in droplets of saliva survives best in indoors and dry conditions. The virus dies quickest in the presence of direct sunlight."

A slide presented by Bryan also recommended moving activities outside. The study was conducted under idealized conditions in a controlled setting. Bryan said, "That in the real world, the virus on a playground surface exposed to direct sunlight would die quickly, but the virus could survive longer in shaded areas."

President Trump commented, "The results vindicate him for his much criticized suggestions that the virus would ebb with the arrival of warm weather. When the surface is outside, it goes very quickly. It dies very quickly with the Sun."

This information is the results of the most recent laboratory testing on the COVID-19 and presented to the public by the United States government.

With that being said, the reality of the disinfecting, purifying, and healing benefits of the sun is not new; it has been accepted as such since ancient times by a multitude of civilizations around the globe. One of the reasons the sun has repeatedly been worshipped as a God for eons.

I want now to relate this wonderful data confirmed by Homeland Security with historical documentation I sourced from the public domain about the practices developed for a group of sailors who had fallen deathly ill while aboard their vessels in the harbor of East Boston in 1918. Recent scholarship suggested that there were three waves of an extremely infectious virus called the Spanish flu between 1918 and 1919. The first wave hit and caused relatively few fatalities. The second wave was in a different manner. The virus spread around the world, like a wildfire spreading the disease in a brief period of a few months, and the results were disastrous. At least half of a million people in the United States succumbed to the virus seemingly in days.

So many deaths occurred in Boston, Massachusetts; the hospitals experienced an overwhelming amount of infected dead bodies that they had the cadavers stored in piles beneath the hospitals while awaiting trucks to haul them away for safe disposal to keep from further contamination of the epidemic to the healthy.

The hospitals became severely overcrowded, and to add to the problems, there were over five thousand merchant marine sailors, trapped aboard their vessels while anchored in the local harbor. There were 1,200 of the crew members had already been officially diagnosed with the deadly Spanish flu and were dying in the tight confines of their ships as the virus spread rapidly in the close quarters.

The Massachusetts State Guard was called in to build a temporary facility to facilitate 351 of the stricken sailors at Corey Hill in Brookline near Boston. An open-air hospital was constructed called Brooks Camp.

At this time in history, there were few medicines and antibiotics had not been invented yet that could aid the suffering's immune systems to help them overcome the fast killing pandemic. The treatment protocol of the day was to make the infected as comfortable as possible, allowing their immune systems to help them recover or to die.

Following reading this data, I could easily see that same pattern in how the UK medical protocols had been designed and how they were implemented. They seemed much more concerned about the health and care of the sailors then than the care with my fiancé.

The camp was only open for thirty days, and the facility only suffered thirty-six deaths of the ill-fated sailors, which was a significant reduction of deaths compared to the hospital environments.

The protocol for the treatment of the sailors at Brooks Camp was all done outdoors in tents with a maximum amount of sunshine and outside air day and night. When the weather was suitable, the sailors were removed from their tents and placed on stretchers outside in the direct sunlight.

Major Thomas Harrington, acting as the medical officer in charge of the facility, took a strong interest to the men and studied each one learning their history and discovered that the most ill had been aboard in the vessels in the most confined spaces that had poor ventilation. The major had little resources to treat the men and decided to make certain things: They were well fed, warmed to strengthen their immune systems with plenty of fresh air and direct sunlight.

Following the closing of Brooks Camp and examining the statistics between the open-air hospital and the existing hospitals determined the average fatality rate was 40 percent at the hospitals, but at Camp Brooks was reduced to 13 percent—a remarkable testament to the healing powers of sunlight and fresh air. When the Brooks Camp data was released to the public, it included this statement: "The efficacy of open-air treatment has been absolutely proven, and one only has to try it to discover its value."

After the third wave of Spanish flu circumnavigated the globe, it had been estimated that as many as fifty to one hundred million people lost their lives to this killer pandemic. It is accepted by all researchers since that period that an accurate account of how many died during those two years will never be known for sure because of poor accounting, communication and the sheer number of primitive cultures that existed at the time that had no contact with the civilized world. It is also accepted that some of these isolated communities suffered a 100 percent fatalities rate, killing the entire communities.

While today, in a short term, we do not have any statistical data gathered to support the Brook's findings from the fresh air and sunlight treatment system for flu-type viruses, particularly the COVID-19; we must take into consideration that a threat of a second wave of the pandemic has to be taken seriously.

It is my opinion based on my life experiences with the sun that every opportunity should be examined as a method to protect and improve our immune systems in order to develop the strongest and best immune system we can own to provide the greatest protection to any future viruses and attacks against our health.

With that being said, I would like to conclude my earlier comment about why I may have infected Heidi with the coronavirus and possibly at least one other person as well.

On January 8, 2020, I was scheduled to leave London via Heathrow Airport and return to the States following a two-month visit with Heidi at her home. I arrived at Heathrow and went through the customary procedures and was seated on the plane. The plane went about the typical preflight checks, and we taxied down the runway preparing for takeoff. As we waited for our turn to take off, the captain came on the intercom and announced there was a medical emergency on the plane, and we had to return back to the terminal delaying our flight until this matter was resolved.

Once we taxied back to the terminal, in a matter of minutes, five rescue personnel came on board the plane, and they all walked past me, carrying their equipment. I was sitting in the aisle seat, so I had to do the lean to give them more room for the tight confines to lug their gear. They went past me about four rows behind me and attended to a man who was also sitting in an aisle seat same as me. Guessing I would say they attended to this gentleman approximately from thirty to forty-five minutes. Then the rescue crew with the man between them walked past me once again and deplaned. This was the first time I could see the man at close range and identified him as a white man in his forties. He was walking on his own reconnaissance without assistance.

In total, the time delay was over one and half hours, and we never heard any comments from the captain as to the circumstances surrounding this incident. We once again taxied down the runway and had a successful takeoff.

It is a long flight to Atlanta from London, and at some point, into the trip, I experienced an incident I still cannot explain. As if I had been stabbed in the abdomen, suddenly I found myself in excruciating pain and bent forward in my seat, trying to relieve the intense pain. In a relatively short period, the pain subsided, and I returned to reading a book Heidi had loaned me for the trip.

It was an exhausting trip, and finally after a layover and second connecting flight, making my way to Norfolk and getting an Uber, I arrived at my floating abode the sea spirit and immediately found my way to the master stateroom and fell into a deep sleep.

The next morning, I awoke and felt as if I had been runover by a bus. I suffered from severe fatigue and found it very difficult to get out of bed. I believed at the time I was experiencing the worst case of jet-lag I had ever experienced in my fifty years of flying. The fatigue and lack of motivation to get out of bed continued, and I was sleeping twelve to fourteen hours a day and night, taking naps and having to force myself to eat.

Frequently, Heidi and I communicated about me feeling so bad, and I would always say, "I was lovesick." We would always laugh.

It was a very special circumstance for me to have felt so bad for so long. Historically, I have not been sick in years, no colds, flus, or allergies. I am fit and healthy and have bragged many times about how strong my immune system was. For over two weeks I suffered many symptoms that you could find now on a standard COVID-19 symptoms list, but for me it was the tremendous fatigue and lack of motivation that really took the life out of me.

One afternoon, while walking up to the marina office to get my mail, I ran into a neighbor I had spoken to and been in his company several times since my return, and he had suddenly been stricken severely ill. I spoke to him the day before he was admitted into the local hospital with an infected lung disease, diagnosed by his doctors during a three-week stay in the hospital including a period in critical care. When I eventually heard his diagnosis, I thought it was very odd for a young healthy man who doesn't smoke.

Heidi and I had made plans for her to fly to America for a two-week visit, and we would return to London together to meet friends for a one-week research adventure to Malta. She arrived ironically on January 29—the very same day President Trump launched the White House Coronavirus Task Force.

One week of her visit, she became suddenly ill; and after two days sick in bed, I made arrangements to get her some medical care. The attending physician, following an exam, prescribed Heidi a number of prescription drugs—at least, one was a series of antibiotics. She began to feel better but never did feel very well; she often complained "that her immune system was under attack" and said "she felt like she had an inflammation caused by a cytokines attack."

Heidi, having been a professional massage therapist for years, has great knowledge about medical science. She had to explain to me what a cytokine was, and in short, it is a form of protein that causes inflammation to such an extent that it weakens the immune system. Since learning this, I also discovered that is one of the attacks the coronavirus uses also.

We made our way satisfactorily to London and then preceded for a week in Malta. Heidi was never at 100 percent, and I admire her tenacity for keeping the entire trip going; she was on medication.

During our seven days in Malta, which happens to be located off the "tip of the boot" of the Italian Peninsula, was the time when Italy went into a total lockdown due to the spread of the coronavirus and were even anchoring some of their navy vessels in the Malta harbor. We were in the middle of a whirlwind research tour with plans to return to London for a few days before heading for a scheduled two weeks to Cairo, Egypt, to further our research on the Giza pyramids.

Once we had arrived at Heidi's residence, the increasing amount of information about the coronavirus spreading worldwide was extremely unsettling to us; and we became concerned that if we continued on to Egypt, we could find ourselves stuck in Egypt during a pandemic lockdown, becoming prisoners in a foreign land with no support systems.

After much deliberation and discussion, we decided to cancel our plans at great expense; and since I had some business appointments scheduled in the America, I made arrangements to fly back to the States immediately to avoid becoming locked down in London adding more cost to our losses.

It turned out our intuition was correct. During our reserved time in Egypt, the country went into lockdown, and we prevented ourselves from being in a very bad situation. Also, soon afterward, the UK went into lockdown as well, and I would have been stranded there. So in hindsight, all our decisions were right on target but costly in money, and today it has been almost three months since I have seen Heidi. I miss her so much.

To live separated in different countries with the Atlantic Ocean between us, and to be in love during a global pandemic is no fun. It was shortly after I left London, Heidi, having completed her round of antibiotics from the US, her health deteriorated, and she fell more seriously ill.

I never was tested for the coronavirus, nor was Heidi or my friend who finally recovered and released from the hospital, following a terrible ordeal.

My thoughts can only wonder about the gentleman who delayed the flight at Heathrow and why he was escorted off the plane. I have to ask myself, Had he just returned from China? That answer most likely will never be known.

In closing, I would like to add that once Heidi completed her fourteen days of quarantine, she had improved. However, still under government lockdown and interesting enough, London was experiencing historical record breaking warm sunny temperatures, and Heidi decided to sunbathe daily as often as she could in her own garden.

I am happy to report my Heidi has made a great recovery and is at 100 percent and has done very well. I cannot wait to see her soon.

CHAPTER 2

GENERAL INFORMATION ABOUT THE SUN

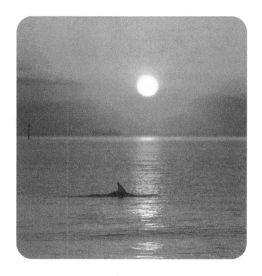

Let's go over some general information about our powerful star that provides humankind light and provides all the components for life here on Earth, the Sun.

The sun is the biggest planet in our planetary system. The sun comprises 99.8 percent of the weight of all our planets combined. The sun continuously sends fireballs which are fifty thousand kilometers long and nine thousand kilometers wide and injects them toward earth some two hundred thousand kilometers.

The mass of the sun is some three hundred twenty-three thousand times the mass of the earth. It has extremely high surface temperatures and goes on producing immense amounts of energy. The sun is in fact a huge ball of gas with hydrogen forming by far its most abundant constituent. Temperatures at its surface is some five thousand five hundred degrees Celsius at its core, where the material is still gaseous though almost a hundred sixty times the density of water. There the temperature approaches approximately fifteen million degrees Celsius.

The sun transmits to each square centimeter of the surface of the earth every minute an amount of heat energy of about two calories, which is enough to raise the temperature of two grams of water one degree Celsius.

Sunlight is composed of many different forms of energy. This energy is transmitted as electromagnetic waves. These waves vary in length from .00001 of a nanometer (for cosmic rays, a nanometer is 1/1,000,000,000 of a meter) to about five thousand kilometers or three thousand one hundred miles for electric waves. This is an incredible wide range of energy radiations for one single source to produce. Not all the rays make it to earth's surface and our bodies. The atmosphere around the earth protects us from absorbing all these numerous wavelengths.

The human eye can only see a fraction of the electromagnetic spectrum that penetrates the atmospheres protection amounting to a fraction of 1 percent. Including in this 1 percent is ultraviolet and infrared. It is the ultraviolet sunlight that has been the most biologically active and the most controversial, and it has been mostly filtered out of our lives removing valuable minerals and chemicals that allows our bodies to properly metabolize.

The eternal nature of the sun and its deep link between the cosmic sun and the sun element or the soul within every human individual. It is the primal cause of our universe and its cycles of manifestations and annihilations.

Therefore, the sun is the soul of our universe.

I want to offer another perspective on an often misunderstood concept.

Everything on the earth owes its very existence to the sun, our source for light, including life itself.

Looking from a spiritual relationship, I want to compare man's association to the sun. When we speak of the holy trinity, we speak from a religious perspective, put forth by the Christian faith in the western world—the Father, the Son, and the Holy Spirit.

We are taught early on as children that God created the sun, giving us light and, therefore, giving us existence. One of the first passages from the Old Testament says, "[F]rom out of the darkness, God spoke and there was light."

When we think of man and his direct relationship to the Holy Trinity, he has none, really. Dogma has made the Holy Trinity separate, put on display as a choice, a spiritual decision, much like an item at the grocery store placed on a shelf that you can look at, decide if you like it or not, or if it will provide you with your desire, determine if it's worth the price, and you get my point—not associated with man in the least little bit.

So let us examine and compare man's direct relationship with the sun and how we are extensions of that sun's light, including how we are designed to interface our life force with it, to be able to absorb, utilize, and transform it.

If we think of light entering a prism, we know the prism is a triangular-shaped object with three sides. This is what occurs when a single wave band of the sun's white light enters this three-sided prism: the light then is refracted and emits the seven colors that compose a complete beautiful rainbow.

Therefore, from a numerical perspective, one wave band of light enters the three-sided prism creating the seven colors of the rainbow.

$$1 = 3 = 7$$

We must therefore question, if God is the operator of the universe and uses his power of command (will), then he commands the sun, which he created with his voice, to send its light to the prism of man.

If true and with the understanding that man is also a composite of that light produced by the sun, he is the receiver of light, exactly like the prism.

Therefore, this trinity and prism of man being the equal has to be presented this way: once man has sought and discovered truth, then develops the skills to integrate his three sides—the mind, the heart and the will—this being the trinity of man (#3), the prism, this is what happens.

The single wave of white light from the sun (1) enters the prism of man (3), and man, if he is clear and pure, then emits into the world for all to share the full spectrum and splendor of the rainbow (7).

We all have heard our entire lives when we speak of someone so positively charged, we say he is bright as the sun. Again it requires man to have a direct relationship with the sun.

I offer *Canticle of the Sun*, written by Saint Francis, to collaborate my comments.

"Praise to You O Lord our God, for all your creatures, especially our dear Brother Sun, Who is the day through whom You give us light. Fair is he, in splendor radiant, Of You, Most High, he bears the likeness."

Chapter 3

Overview of Experiments

Initially, before I began to sungaze, I researched thoroughly and discovered that there were a number of ancient methods of sungazing. Sorting through all the ancient techniques I could locate information on, I discovered one that was superior to everything else I examined. The method was ancient and had been revived from a Jain Indian religion that is still practicing sungazing today.

I learned of a gentleman from India, and I decided to utilize his method as one of the Jain's most prized sons, Hira Ratan Manek, had organized. He had been raised in the Jain religion (a sungazing cult, still today) which is a branch of Hinduism religion. HRM, he likes to be called, is a seventy-plus year old man who, at the age of twenty-five years old, began his study of ancient sungazing techniques. Coming from a prominent family, he had the luxury and the contacts to be able to speak with people most of us would never meet that had access to ancient text and information pertaining to sungazing.

HRM took the opportunity to meet with the people who were trusted with this extraordinary information and ancient wisdom. Coming from an affluent family, only someone with his prestige could afford these meetings.

HRM claims he spent twenty-five years of his life researching the ancient art of sungazing. During this time, he said he took all the information he had obtained and compiled a systematic approach to sungazing which he then experimented with, on his own for five additional years. Hira named his method the HRM Protocol, which provides a very detailed and safe approach, from how to begin sungazing, up to the end when you reach the ability to gaze for forty-four minutes' duration.

On March 1, 2014, I began my sungazing experiment using Hira's "HRM protocol," which he advertised as a very detailed and safe method to begin sungazing.

In hindsight now that I have successfully completed these experiments, which I documented in journals and drawings of my visions, I can look back and reflect with an experienced hands-on approach. This allows me the opportunity to offer a different perspective on sungazing, much better than before I started.

Prior to my beginning of HRM's protocol, I had watched a number of videos and studied his simple method outlined in his free e-book titled *Living on Sunlight*, which details his methods in a simple three-phase cyclic program.

Over the next twelve months, I spent two hundred sixty days, totaling ninety hours of documented naked-eyed staring at the sun. It required most of twelve months aggressive pursuit to complete HRM's Protocol where I gained the ability training myself to be able to stare for a forty-five-minute duration.

(Note: while his program suggests forty-four minutes, I added an additional minute which is acceptable because some people's systems are slightly different and results vary a bit.)

From the start of the program, I was determined to follow his recommendations as closely as possible. With respect to his wisdom and in hindsight, I'm happy to admit I did so.

It was once I completed his program that I reviewed my progress, and one big factor physically for me was a significant improvement in my vision.

Prior to starting to sungaze, for several years I had visited the same eye doctor who had diagnosed me early on with having cataracts, and his recommendation was to consider at some point in the future having eye lens replacement surgery to correct my vision issues.

One of the most common symptoms related to having been electrocuted is the accelerated growth of cataracts on the lenses of the eyes. Plus I had been active as a trained metal welder for forty years.

So I began to research the different methods and companies that provided that service. I ended up going to one of the newest companies whose only service is Lasik surgery. I made an appointment with them and experienced a barrage of eye examinations using the most advance computer analysis available at that time. Their final diagnosis based on their testing was I had significant cataracts on both eyes that required lens replacement.

I now had two eye experts who agreed that I had vision issues related to cataracts.

Both of these diagnoses were from years to months before my interest in sungazing developed, and I continued on with life, changing my prescription glasses routinely as needed.

Once I had been sungazing for some time, I did a lecture on another topic about my near-death experience from electrocution and I mentioned the injuries I had suffered and one was the accelerated growth of cataracts on my eyes. I explained I had been sungazing, experimenting in an attempt to correct the problem. In the audience that day was another eye doctor who was fascinated by my comments, and he approached me afterwards with many questions. We began a fast relationship where soon after my lecture, I made an appointment and visited his offices in another local.

He did a full eye examination which included mapping my cataracts by drawing on paper. His final diagnosis, now the third, was I needed lens replacement surgery.

I explained to him my current research on sungazing had discovered positive results of vision improvement, and I wanted to complete this experiment using the HRM method and witness the results, good or bad. If the sungazing proved itself a failure, I would then pursue the necessary corrective surgery.

Returning to my previous comment about the improvements I had in my vision after twelve months of successful sungazing, I then decided to do an independent first-of-its-kind experiment that went way beyond the HRM Protocol and do another sungazing experiment that ended up lasting for seven more months, with each gaze at forty-five-minute duration.

So beginning March 1, 2015, exactly one year from beginning the HRM Protocol, I went rogue.

I was convinced that my vision improvements were in part from the shrinking of the cataracts on my eyes. The reason I felt so strongly to attempt this unreasonable technique was often the morning following a sungazing session, my eyes would contain a crusty debris that had to be removed each time.

I felt confident, and I had an optometrist I was in regular communication with about the progress of my experiments.

The additional gaze time over the next seven months increased my totals to nineteen months long, three hundred forty-four days sungazing, adding an additional sixty-three hours now totaling one hundred fifty-three incredible hours accumulated while staring naked eyed at the sun.

When I read this, I can still hear my mother saying, "Never stare at the sun. It will make you go blind."

The results of my second experiment led me to follow up with my original long-term optometrist for prescription for lens replacement. I chose him because of the insurance provider network I was enrolled with. The eye surgeon's exam for surgery did not go as I expected.

My intentions to write this volume was never to provide a "how to sungaze" step-by-step method book on proper sungazing procedures—why? Because I see no value in any changes to HRM's Protocol.

I would rather describe *Addicted to the Sun* as a hands-on review of the process focused on sharing an intimate record of the personal experiences and benefits one might encounter that I detail from my revealing journals.

The major influences causing significant changes in your daily lifestyle happens as a result during the transition in your anatomical processes. Sungazing naturally adjusts your body to process (1) the sudden increase on information, (2) the gradual ability to tolerate the increase in intensity, (3) thus gaining the skill to be able to process the form of proton light energy efficiently.

Over the required time to complete the program, your body literally attunes to the frequency of the sun. In today's world, the typical human has lost that connection to the sun, being unfamiliar with having a positive relationship with it, but it is simple to reset that connection. That switch can be turned on.

Assimilating this energy and converting it to caloric substance to be used as fuel for the body is within most grasp. I found it easy, safe, and free. You will get no argument from me to disagree with Hira.

One of the things that I stumbled upon at around twenty minutes of ability to stare at the sun was the reduction of hunger pangs, which developed into a lack of desire to eat. I lost all cravings for the foods I loved. The second thing was when I ate, I lost the sensation of satiation, never feeling that fullness and the need to stop. I do feel the volume of food it makes in consuming, but the full gage is non-functional now.

I'm also including as an addendum to my two sungazing experiments my experience of going ninety days as a non-eater. That is being able to use the sun as my primary food source, allowing me to calorically sustain myself from the Sun.

Beginning on December 5, 2016, I decided to experiment and see if my body was attuned to the sun's frequencies sufficiently enough to live without eating food. At that time, my only concern was the season of the year and the astronomical fact that the sun was moving further away from the geographical location I resided.

I already knew, from my experiments, this season phase shift would have a huge impact on the quality or intensity that the sun could provide. I was aware that my self-dedicated food source would be at his weakest cycle and may not be able to provide me with the vitamins, minerals, and building-block amino acids of proteins to meet my basic requirements.

As I did with sungazing, I approached the non-eating experiment by engaging the knowledge and resources of my personal physician, who at my request on day seventy-five, performed a physical exam complete with blood work monitoring my blood chemistry with particular attention placed on proteins levels.

With this in mind, I began this journey of trying to live a normal life without eating food. I never had a firm grasp how long I would go without eating or when I would take that first bite of solid food again in the future.

I did follow experienced breatharian recommendations learned from reading and research.

Without too many details on this wild journey, I do want to say the first stage to know if your body is ready to stop eating is to do a three-day fast. If you never feel hungry during those days, you are ready for longer fast.

Another addition to this volume is to provide my recipe for rainbow water, as I call it. It is all I have consumed in seven years. When my discoveries of how the pyramid systems worked on the Giza Plateau, I replicated the methods the ancients created that allowed for crops to grow to abundance in the desert sand. This water formula begins as distilled and takes two days to create, but it is high in energy calories. Most people don't understand how the energy of the sun creates our nutrition system nor do they understand that regardless of what foods you eat, none of it ever enters into the blood stream; it is an energy exchange only. I'll explain this along the way.

I hope you enjoy the information I have put in print as much as I enjoyed learning it firsthand. I look at these experiments as some of the greatest events of my lifetime.

Chapter 4

Some Ancient History/Tesla's Sungazing Experience

We know that many ancient cultures and civilizations held the sun in high regard.

The Egyptians expanded their relationship with the sun well beyond the scope or concept of "sun worship." Sun worship was a way of life for those with status, prestige, and authority.

All the greatest spiritual masters, sages, and teachers through the ages knew that the physical sun was a gateway to another world. They also believed there was a second star also, another sun, and was hidden in the brilliance of our own sun, as it shines brightest and significant because of its closer proximity to earth.

My years of independent research has led me to believe without a doubt the hidden second star they were referencing was Sirius, which is a part of the Orion constellation, and is known as the Dog Star. Sirius dwarfs our sun in immensity, and many ancient civilizations considered Sirius the mother of our sun.

While these scenarios create a binary solar system, our sun being positive masculine energy, Sirius is the opposite with negative feminine energy. Our universal suns the true yin/yang of our cosmic bipolar energy system.

The ancients also understood that sunlight was the conveyer of expanding intelligence and had the ability to increase information capacity and availability. They believed the sun was not only the source of life on earth, but it could unlock latent, spiritual faculties within the human mind. This occurred by what they believed were sacred factors, which streamed into the physical world from heavenly or divine realms above.

These were the teachings of the great masters, on which noble religions and philosophies are founded, still today. Some of these great masters include Menkaure, Moses, Aaron, Jesus, Buddha, Krishna, Viracocha, Quetzalcoatl, Socrates, Plato, Akhenaten, Confucius, Lao Tzu, and many others.

The sun offers 100 percent sustenance for man to survive as a non-eater, or breatharian, obtaining his entire mineral, vitamin, and energy calories necessary to thrive and live a healthy and lengthy life-time directly from that source, the sun.

In 1899, Nikola Tesla was interviewed by John Smith, a jour-nalist for *Immortality Magazine*. It is a famous interview known today as the "Everything is the Light" interview. It took place in Colorado Springs, Colorado, where Tesla had constructed a lab, and his experiments with lightning and early designs on what became the Wardenclyffe Tower he constructed and tested in Long Island, New York, as his main focus.

During the interview, Tesla's perspectives and demeanor were expressed numerous times when speaking of sunlight. It is apparent that Tesla's mood and attitude, which was projected during the inter-view, reflected a man who was comfortable, a man who felt at home, and he was. Compared to other interviews I've read given by Tesla, this article shows a side of Tesla which reflects who Tesla was—as himself.

Tesla had been living in Colorado for some time after moving his lab from New York City to Colorado Springs. He was having the time of his life—solitude, nature, and natural electricity. Tesla had become so comfortable living in Colorado and so familiar with the frequent lightning storms that he gave the recurring lightning bolts individual names. Some of them he called by family names.

During the interview, Tesla questioned Mr. Smith, asking, "Do you know how I discovered the rotating magnetic field, induc-tion motor, which made me famous, when I was twenty-six?" Tesla answered his own question.

"One summer in Budapest, I watched the sunset with my friend Sigetijem. Thousands of fire were turning around and thousands of flaming colors. I remembered Faust and recited his verses, and then as if a fog, I saw a spinning magnetic field, and induction motor. I saw them in the sun!"

This is the second time I have read an interview between Tesla and another journalist where he speaks of this same incident and his discovery of alternating current (AC) and how it came about during the interactions with his friend while they were working together in Budapest. Tesla also tells the same story in his autobiography.

I share more collaborative information that supports Tesla's lifestyle as a sungazer as well as his being a non-eater in the later years of his life at the end of the experiments.

Viktor Schauberger, an Austrian naturalist, inventor, philosopher, and author writing numerous books, is well known as the "Water Wizard." He claims his discoveries and unconventional understandings of physics and mathematics were made by dispatching "free consciousness into those places where the eyes cannot see… the Akosha." He was firm in his beliefs that his method was the only way to make practical discoveries, discounting those that felt the discoveries were foolish conjecture.

Walter, his son, became an engineer and spent his life creating mathematical formulas and experiments to prove his father's theories. He also created and published a scientific magazine, *Implosion Magazine*, with much of his findings.

In my research prior to my non-eating experiment, I used some of Walter's formulas as well as other proven scientific data to create a method to understand the sun's energy on the earth and creating an energy grid system of how the sun's energy stream influences the human.

Once I completed the HRM protocol of gaining the ability to stare naked-eyed at the sun for forty-four minutes duration, for some reason, I decided I would continue increasing my time to forty-five minutes and then gaze for duration for an undetermined time. Intuition perhaps?

I also decided to extend my extended gaze of forty-five minutes in terms of a timeframe till the end of September 2015, thus adding seven more months. I felt since my time gazing had been maximized in the month of March, I had spent my longest gazes of my experiment during the colder months of the year when the sun was its weakest intensity. I had another inclination, a feeling again, at that time that I was having some success with cataract removal by gazing. I had already suspected it was not the just the light improving the cataract sloughing, it was the temperature of the sun in combination with the light. I felt it necessary to be able to utilize the sun's intensity at its maximum, which meant gazing during the summer months.

As of September 30, I had gazed nineteen months straight. Since March 1, 2015, I have gazed eighty-four times, all but a few were for the total timeframe of forty-five minutes.

This adds an additional sixty-three hours of sungazing to my already accumulated time of ninety hours, total one hundred fifty-three hours, and a total of three hundred forty-four days of active gazing experiences for the grand total for both sungazing experiments.

CHAPTER 5

HIGHLIGHTS OF THE **HRM** PROTOCOL

Let us discuss the method now. Below is the information available of Hira's great Surya yoga (sungazing) system:

The HRM Protocol (free e-book, pdf download) in the *Living on Sunlight: The Art and Science of Sun Gazing,* as taught by Hira Ratan Manek, HRM, compiled and edited by Vina Parmar, MBA.

HRM can be contacted at hiraratanmanek@yahoo.com and on his website www.solarhealing.com.

The brief excerpts I share in this text are direct from Hira's writings and his lectures. I gratefully give him his due and much deserved credit respect to all his work, all the years research, and taking the risk himself personally to test the various methods of sungazing, compiling a safe sungazing protocol that is simple, easy, and free. We all should be grateful for his contributions.

In my direct correspondence with him, he was generous and enthusiastic about me lecturing and writing about his method, saying to me, "Tell the world."

This is my attempt to share his message.

HRM, as he prefers to be called, says, "We have a supercomputer in our bodies which is our brain." He calls it the "brainutor."

The brain is the more powerful than the most advanced supercomputer known today. Each and every one of us has innumerable talents and infinite, inherent powers given to us by nature. We should never underestimate ourselves. If we make use of these powers, we can take our selves to great levels.

Unfortunately, these powers are programmed in a part of the brain which is largely dormant and unused. Medical science says we only use about 5 to 7 percent of our brain. Geniuses, like Einstein, used 32 percent of his brain.

In order to operate the brain effectively, we need to activate it. Sun energy is the power source for the human brain. This sun energy can enter and leave the human body. It can enter the brain through only one organ—the eye. The eyes are the sun's entry doors to the brain, also called "windows of the soul."

Recent scientific research has revealed the human eye has many more functions than just sight.

The eye is a complex organ containing about five billion different parts.

HRM says, "The rainbow is not in the sky, it's in the eye. The seven colors of the Sun are only a reflection of what is in the eye. We can create a rainbow any time we want."

(Note: I routinely see the rainbow colors surrounding and being emitted from the sun. A color I would have not thought to see as the most abundant is the color magenta.)

The eye can receive the entire spectrum of sunlight; it is like having a glass window. Since eyes are very delicate, we must protect them and use them in ways that will not damage them. Hysteria and paranoia of the past, such as "Don't stare at the sun," "The sun causes cancer," and teachings and ideas which are false.

The more you stay away from the nature, the more you risk illness.

Also, the absence from sunlight heavily supports the global corporate community.

There are definite ways, which are foolproof and safe ways, to get the benefits of nature without exposing ourselves to its adverse effects.

In the HRM Protocol, Hira instructs, the very first gaze, to make certain, that there are two times a day, that are absolutely safe to stare at the sun with naked eyes. There is a timeframe, forty-five minutes at sunrise and forty-five minutes at sunset, that the UV conditions are zero.

HRM recommends beginning sungazing with a ten-second gaze for the very first time, and each gaze following the first gaze to add an additional ten seconds to the first gaze. An example would be first gaze ten seconds, second gaze twenty seconds, third gaze thirty seconds, and see how simple it is.

Hira also claims that it that it should take a time period of nine months to complete his program.

(Note: However, in my experience—and I was very aggressive with my endeavor to complete this program in the nine-month timeframe— weather conditions would have to be perfect every day.)

To make comment on my experiences, my total hours to complete the HRM Protocol went this way:

As I stated earlier, I was very tenacious and very aggressive with my time to gaze; I made it a high priority in my day. Many days I gazed twice—sunrise and sunset because of cloudy or unfavorable conditions in the morning. I would take the two times and add them together to fulfill the required amount for that day. For example, when I was at ten minutes total time, if I could only gaze three minutes at sunrise and the afternoon sky cleared, I would gaze the seven minutes I couldn't in the morning. I found this an acceptable method, and then the next gaze time I would add the standard ten seconds.

During the winter months, I spent my mornings barefoot in freezing cold temperatures, standing in the sand, cold wind off the Atlantic blowing in my face, anxiously waiting for the sun to rise up out of the great Atlantic Ocean.

I completed the HRM Protocol toward the end of February 2015, almost a year exactly from when I began on March 1, 2014.

I concluded I had successfully stared at the sun for total collected time of ninety hours active sungazing to be able to stare at the sun, naked-eyed, for forty-five minutes duration.

I gazed two hundred sixty days out of three hundred sixty, completing the HRM Protocol just five days shy of one year.

I learned as you sungaze, in the time your eyes adjust, the rods and cones of the eyes become attuned to the intensity of the sun. For me, my eyes were very sensitive to any type of light because of the damages the electricity caused to my optic nerve. I wore sunglasses all the time, even in darkness. I had all but stopped driving at night because the scattered headlight glare of the cars blinded me so, even with sunglasses on.

When I first began ten seconds for the first gaze, the tears poured from my eyes as if I was peeling a really strong onion.

With sungazing, it's one of those things like riding a bicycle; you talk to people who have never ridden all you want and tell them how it works and even demonstrate how to do it, but they have to actually try for themselves before they can appreciate exactly what it is they have to do. The difference with sungazing is it is much simpler.

Hira states that,

> All illnesses begin with defective neurons in the brain which eventually cause physical problems in the body. The Sun does heal and generates new neurons and gray matter in the brain, even after the age of 50 when neuron depletion accelerates. Sungazing can halt this negative progression and increase the Neuron community.

He claims that the history of sungazing is ancient, and many civilizations practiced. Some are the Ariens, the Mongolians, the Egyptians, the Incas, the Mayans, the Peruvians, the Bulgarians, the Greeks, the Eastern Indians, the Mesopotamians, and the Native American Indians.

Sungazing was originally created on religious beliefs and, now today in modern times, attitudes will eventually change and sungazing will one day be considered high-tech.

Sungazing has been practiced throughout the existence of humankind throughout the world, up to the last few thousand years.

Hira also states,

> [T]he sun can never harm you if used properly, also, walking barefoot on the earth is

mentally healthful, practicing mentally peaceful walking changes the brain and all health problems then cured. Your hidden divine and true nature then come to the surface. Depression, Schizophrenia, and phobias can be healed, and all hunger disappears.

By the time you reach this point, your body has developed mechanisms to depend on energy directly from the sun. You do not control hunger, it just disappears, and your external bad habits turn into external good habits. You develop the ability to be in constant meditation with your eyes open fully conscious of your surroundings.

Walking barefoot in addition opens more of the brain and stimulates the pineal gland. The walking of barefoot in the sand creates a reflexology treatment for the toes, energizes the nerve endings, and sends that information linking it to certain parts of the endocrine system. Attuning your energy frequencies to the sun brings complete wellness in the mind, body, and spirit. The powerful energies that accompany the light activate the dormant areas of the brain.

Sungazing and walking barefoot or Earth-walking used to be for Pharaohs, kings, queens, high priests, and high priestesses only. Lord Mahavir of the Jain religion is like the Buddha of the Jain religion.

HRM claims that for years he suffered from depression and sleeplessness was cured by sungazing. Hira does not eat food, he only drinks boiled distilled water from 11:00 a.m. to 4:00 p.m. each day.

He claims he began sungazing at the age of fifty, beginning his research at twenty-five, and researched for thirty years total. At age seventy-three, he was studied by NASA, and some of their investigative findings determined his brain cells were still growing and his pineal gland is enlarged and measured three times the normal size.

(Note: The ancient Indians believed dying occurs of the physical body when the pineal gland (the seat of the soul) atrophies and shrinks until it shrivels to where it is no longer function. It is the time when physical death occurs, and the light body, the soul, then escapes from the body through the eyes.)

There are unproven claims that the sun can heal multiple sclerosis. It can and does decrease the appetite, and there is an immediate, increase in the body's energy levels. The accelerated energy levels are subsidized by including solar charged water and sunbathing.

Modern science and pharmaceutical companies have instilled fear into the average citizen with regards to the sun when in reality, the longer you abstain from the light, the more illness you will suffer.

Freedom cannot exist with dependence on others. You have to take control for your own personal health and safety.

Sungazing has been shown to decrease the symptoms of dementia, Alzheimer's, and Parkinson's diseases. The sun extinguishes and removes all stress so the brain can relax. Once the brain has relaxed and become balanced, the neurons can heal and regenerate.,

Once you have completed the HRM Protocol and your sungazing has reached forty-four minutes, your mood will not be influenced by any of the planets moon cycles or astrological events. Nothing can really disturb you, even the reading of astrology can cease because the planetary influences have been removed.

(Note: it was my experience that while these natural cosmic influences may not influence your behavior, if you are a sensitive and aware of these influences, you will still be able to feel them. However, I do agree you will not be influenced by them because you are vibrating at a higher frequency.)

The pineal gland also known as the seat of the soul and will enlarge naturally extending your life span. The soul becomes comfortable with its own skin. Today, over eighteen thousand researchers are now studying the pineal gland's functions more than any time in history. Up until recent years, the pineal gland was a mystery. No one really understood the pineal gland, and it didn't appear to have any major importance. It was usually overlooked when it came to brain research.

Sungazing can cause the spine to straighten and spinal nerves to reconnect. Bone deterioration decreases and growth is regenerated. The sun can heal damaged teeth because sunlight makes vitamin D, and vitamin D makes calcium. Even individuals that are blind can receive 10 percent benefit themselves from sungazing with their eyelids closed because the receptors in their eyes are damaged so even they can get some benefit from the sun.

The wearing of sunglasses full time is not recommended. Sunglasses should be used when walking on the beach and driving one's car to eliminate damaging glare. Sunglasses should also be worn for boating on saltwater and participating in snow events such as downhill skiing or sledding. Due to the fear of sunlight and corporate marketing campaigns, 90 percent of all people who constantly wear sunglasses have insomnia or sleep=related maladies.

Barefoot walking in the sand or in the dirt is good for obesity, the eyes, and common stomach ailments. Sungazing has an effect on respiration. As the length of your sungazing increases, your breathing will slow down naturally to ten breaths or below per minute. Also, the sunlight helps to extend life because the ancients believed a human only has an imprint for so many breaths.

All dreams will be eliminated because people who dream are people who are worried or have disturbed minds. Sungazing creates calm meditation around the clock, which eliminates dreams and unbalanced mind. The amount of sleep is reduced with sleeping and adequate length of time, just enough to feel refreshed and free from fatigue. The experienced sungazer will no longer suffer from jetlag.

When you cannot gaze during the two safe gazing zones, you can still accomplish your goal by gazing at noon time in the sun's reflection in fresh water, such as a river or lake. It is a matter of safety and mandatory that the water be fresh clear water and not contain salt. I want to include snow as part of this warning because both are very harmful to the eyes.

Before beginning to sungaze, any type of glasses needs to be removed for safety. Some eyeglass lenses refract the sunlight, so significantly you can use the lenses like a magnifying glass and catch paper on fire. Your eyeglass prescriptions will change frequently as your eyes recover, and sometimes your original vision can return.

(Note: Over time, I noticed myself more observant of my surroundings and environment. I have begun to notice ordinary things for which I formally paid little attention. My awareness sharpened, and I noticed

a lot more activity around me. It is amazing the plethora of information I have received because of increased sensitivity and increased curiosity.)

(Note: this info came from a YouTube video I watched, it is an hour-long lecture-with HRM. He says, "Sungazing for the first three months is for mental health, sungazing in Phase 2, the second three months is for physical health, and sungazing for Phase 3 the third and final three months of the program is for spiritual health and enlightenment.")

Hira also recommended, "Once you complete the program that sungazing is not necessary any longer that the next phase to activate the pineal gland is to walk barefoot in dry sand not wet for forty-five-minute duration." He also said, "Walking in dirt was an excellent way to introduce nutrients, such as bromine, into the body through the souls of the feet." He demonstrated the posture most used to sungaze which is holding hands up with arms bent ninety degrees or parallel to the earth with palms facing toward the sun.

He said that "it did not matter where you sun gazed from as far as location except to not do it on grass, not even to walk bare foot on grass that it depletes the body of energy." He continued saying, "Other than that, anywhere else to sungaze that the difference between the worst and best methods is marginal. Therefore, location is secondary."

From his protocol, he claims that sungazing awakens the dormant resources inside the human brain. He says, "The greatest welfare program for all men is sungazing."

Science has now determined sunlight falls into two categories: safe sunlight is medicine, and intense sunlight is poison.

Safe sunlight for the eyes is 0 to 2 UV and for skin is 2 to 5 UV. However, it could safely be 0 to 5 UV.

Sungazing has been practiced for millennia by all of humankind throughout the world up to the last few thousand years.

HRM says that following nine months of gazing. If you lose desire to eat and can go three days without hunger, you have reached the pinnacle and can stop sungazing and then do barefoot walking.

Chapter 6

Some Comments from Experienced Sungazers

As you are aware, my research and text is only a sample of my guru, Hira Ratan Manek's great work, and I am only giving his recommendations to stress the importance of safety and providing some of his wonderful information. It is mandatory before you begin sungazing to download *Living on Sunlight* and read it thoroughly before your first gaze.

In my research prior to my own experimentation, I also read other people's volumes, who some had followed the HRM Protocol themselves, and they share their own unique perspectives that influenced me as well and I want share some of those. If I am sharing their works, I also highly recommending you read their great contributions as well.

It is good to have others' opinions and positive experiences to develop confidence in attempting to sungaze.

Read *The Earth Was Flat: Insight into the Ancient Practice of Sungazing* by Mason Howe Dwinell, LAC.

Mason Howe Dwinell has a good delivery, and his comments add to the understanding how sungazing works. He says,

> Sungazing can create experiences to stir up the magic that is within every individual. As our subtle energies awaken, we may become aware that there is more to life than meets the eye. And

it is with this awareness that we may begin to taste our limitless potential.

Mr. Dwinell relates a good description of HRM's protocol.

He says, "Cleaning one's food intake with purer foods, vegetarian diet, and increased sungazing time will increase vibrational energy."

Some people may develop issues where they influence electrical equipment such as cellphone batteries going dead after twenty minutes or lose interest in eating food. Many sungazers who were left on the curb by western medicine are enjoying a healthy existence through sungazing. Regardless of cancer, HIV/AIDS, a broken leg, the flu—anything is possible. Sungazing aids in the body, being able to find its energetic equilibrium. There is something rather unique about the sun's energy.

He states,

> I have viewed the sun from just about every-where. I stood on grass, on sand, in mud, in water, on a rock, and on the snow. I have sungazed from a tree, looked through leaves, through fog, and through clouds. I have watched the Sun rise from a plane, a car and a boat. I have sungazed from sea level to 14,000 feet and every-where in between. Picturing myself as a battery, the heavens and earth, north and south poles. Envisioning this way may have enabled me to be anywhere and still benefit from the suns energy.

He confirms HRM's ten-second rule:

> Going faster than 10 seconds offers no benefits, slow and steady as the effects are substantial both mentally and physically. The effects on yourself will have an effect on your friends and your family, any one you meet.

Good advice he offers:

> If you miss some time due to bad weather start back where you left off unless it has been many weeks, months or year. Start back in 5-minute increments a few days in a row and then go up another 5 for a few days till you were at the time you stopped and then go back to 10 seconds a day.

> You must believe that staring into the sun is safe and will cause no harm and you must allow the rods and cones of the eyes adjust as the Sunlight passes through your eyes.

> Some say Sungazing works with the Suns energy following the Optic nerve which stimulates the Pineal Gland. This in turn activates the hypothalamus which governs the endocrine system and other hormones in the body creating ample energy for a human to live.

I really liked this comparison:

> Another idea is comparing photosynthesis to an energetic reaction inside the human. How it works is not as important as the fact that it does work. Embrace it, love it, and utilize it. Better yet expand on it and become present with it so that it becomes yours. Then it becomes yours forever.

> Intention plays a big part with Sungazing as with anything else. Energy follows intent.

(Note: This was very true in my case and why when I reached forty-four minutes, I was surprised I didn't notice any significant difference.

By increasing one minute longer to forty-five minutes, I suddenly felt as if a light switch had been turned on.)

Information I've gathered from multiple sources offer this information that I feel explains the relationship between humans and plants, very well.

The correlation of Sun light between hemoglobin (in blood) and chlorophyll (in plants). Hemoglobin has the same chemical formula and function as chlorophyll, except that hemoglobin has iron (Fe) in its center and chlorophyll has magnesium (Mg) in its.

Therefore, the effects of the Sun on chlorophyll could be related to effects of the Sun on hemoglobin. The link between hemoglobin and chlorophyll and the 44 minutes of blood movement could be insight into the possibilities of Sungazing. Theoretically, we can photo synthesize energy just like a plant. That seems to be as good as an explanation as any.

The 44-minute maximum is explained that it takes 44 minutes for the whole amount of blood in the human body to circulate and pass through the retina in the eyes. The retina is the only place in the body where the sunlight touches blood. (directly or almost directly) the 44-minute time frame is an average and could vary person to person.

(Note: I can say this, and you will read the comments in my daily journal. I could feel the magnetic pull of the sun. It physically pulled me toward it like a flower turning toward the sunlight. At times, I felt as if I may fall flat on my face.)

I would like to take the time now to provide some additional basic systems details about the Retina of the eye that I have found most extraordinary based upon my own individual research.

Sunlight Rays and most artificial light passes through the Lens of the eye, as they enter the eye, which acts similar to a magnifying glass in the way it bends the light and aims it at the rear of the retinal back surface of the eye. The eye gathers as much light as the aperture we call the pupil allows to enter. This adjusted Sunlight is compressed by the Lens and is targeted for three important systems at the rear of the eye: the Macula, the Optic Nerve, and the Central Retinal Blood Vessels.

Before I explain the systems relationship with the Sunlight, I want to include some information I find amazing about the eyes, particularly the Retina.

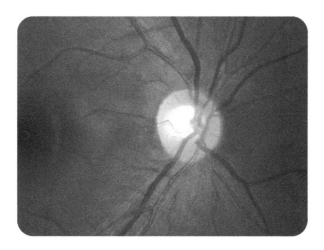

The Retina is one of the most metabolically active tissues in the human body. The Retina consumes oxygen more rapidly than our brains, with such a high oxygen demand the Retina has an extensive vascular network to maintain functionality. Since the highest oxygen demands in the eye are located amongst the photoreceptor's inner segments, this requires a vast network of blood supply, there are two major sources of blood flow that provides the volume necessary. They are the Central Retinal Artery and the Choroidal Blood Vessels, which originate from the Ophthalmic Artery, which enter into the Retina through the Head of the Optic Nerve.

Body Basics: The Eye

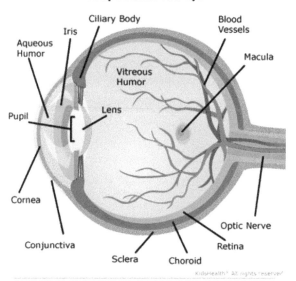

These blood supplies are pumped directly from the heart supply system. The average adult's blood supply system contains a volume of between 1.2 and 1.5 gallons of blood. The Heart circulates this blood through the entire body in a remarkably fast period in less than one minute, actually 45 seconds time frame. In a single day this circulation cycle by our great pump occurs over 100,000 times.

While this blood flow circulates and returns to the heart from most of our organs and muscles at lightning speeds the Retina of the eye is a radical exception. While the intraocular tissues and retinal vessels are similar to those found in our brains, the blood flow through the Retina is auto regulated and experiences very little influence from our bodies Sympathetic Nervous System.

Why is this important? The Sympathetic Nervous System's primary process is to stimulate the body's fight-flight-or-freeze response to external stimuli. Therefore, it primes the body for action, particularly in life threatening situations. It causes the Heart to increase Heart Rate and forces contraction. Also, the bodies organs and numerous systems stop production and send this blood and energy to areas of our body, for instance our legs if we need to run as fast as we can. Because of this, the Retina has been protected from the possibility of a sudden shift of blood pressures with its auto regulated systems, so our vision is not affected. It would be a terrible circumstance if we experienced a threat and were so frightened, we wanted to run to safety as fast as we could and suddenly lost our vision, becoming momentarily blind as a result.

The human body is an incredible machine, perfectly designed and capable to do so much more than modern man today attempts.

Now that I've provided a basic understanding of the operation of the eye, I'd like to explain my Hypothesis on how I believe the virus killing potential of Sunlight may be possible to enter— into the human body. It is my hope to continue research in this regard developing some laboratory testing as well to prove my beliefs.

First, I want to comment on some of the information I detailed earlier in chapter 1 that William N. Bryan presented in response to the Laboratory testing he was overseeing for Homeland Security to the President Trump created White House Coronavirus Task Force.

Bryan claimed and Trump repeated that the Laboratory experiments proved that the Coronavirus was destroyed quickly by exposure to Sunlight.

If we look at how the eye is designed, and we take into consideration that the closest and most direct route that Sunlight can enter into the human body is through the eye.

I have already described how the light enters through the Lens of the eye and is magnified onto the rear of the retina that contains the focusing Macula, the Optic Nerve and the delicate bundle of brain like Retinal arteries.

I mentioned that the heart circulates its oxygenized life-giving blood which includes the fantastic healing powers of our Immune system made up of white blood cells and anti-bodies every 45 seconds throughout the entire body but the eye.

I just explained the autoregulation of the blood supply to the Retina and how it was constant and other researchers had determined that it requires 44 minutes for the entire blood supply to pass through the Retina of the eye. This means that the blood during the same time frame, in the rest of the body will have circulated over 2,000 complete cycles to one for the Retina. This means that the Sunlight will have been focused on these tiny delicate blood vessels the entire time.

My question is this: If Sunlight kills the Coronavirus on the skin or doorknobs or children's playground equipment quickly, how fast can it kill the virus in our blood supply by Sungazing?

There have been instances where people have starred at the Sun all day and been okay. War prisoners forced to stare at sun without harmful effects. They reported to having had head splitting headaches and brilliant spots within their vision for a few days then they began to improve their general health and energy levels were reported as 10-fold.

Once you reach 44 minutes you don't have to Sungaze any longer. You can keep and maintain your electrical charge in many ways. Some folks just meditate and focus on the Anja Chakra (pineal gland). Some walk on bare earth bare foot for 45 minutes to an hour a day. Some can maintain charge just being in the Sun a couple minutes every day and some use unique breathing techniques.

(Note: I have experimented with all these methods and agree 100 percent. There are other methods as well. What I discovered is once you are attuned, there is an abundance of energy to the extent it is very easy to become over stimulated. Energy management becomes a necessary learned technique.)

There is no wrong way to Sungaze. Your senses will change, you will be able to feel the energy differences between certain foods. You will be able to recognize foreign energy. You become much more curious about sensations throughout your body and mind.

Sungazing creates an awareness that you cannot escape. The cleaner your diet the bigger influence the Suns energy has on the bodies' cells. Alcohol, smoking and drugs need to stop.

As your cells increase their over-all health you may find your body reacts negatively to processed foods. You may notice that carbohydrates and starches take longer to digest. As your sensitivities increase you may feel encouraged to eat your last meal of the day earlier in the day. I couldn't eat past 2pm or couldn't get restful sleep. Like having a mini hangover.

As I reached 30 mins of Sungazing you may need less and less sleep. You will experience more vigor and require less sleep. Going from 8 needed hours of sleep to just 4 or 5 hours a night. As your Sungazing time continues you may find yourself not needing as much food, even to the point that you could stop eating altogether. Becoming a Breatharian.

(Note: at twenty-minute duration, I felt a huge decrease in hunger. I went from three meals a day to two effortlessly.)

"Sex is better, childbirth is fine with mothers who breast feed producing plenty of milk. Children of parents who both Sungazed during conception are normal. Wonderful coherent and capable individuals."

I like his comments about his experiences with children:

Yes even children can Sungaze when they are old enough to understand how to Sungaze properly. Interaction with a 10-year old who Sungazed was humbling by their insight and honesty. Without pretense or attempts to impress they simply shared their truth.

Increased Clairvoyance and intuition and astral travel.

(Note: absolutely, the psychic channels are turned on.)
HRM states,

If we can control our wants, our hungers, we can control our fate and happiness. The pinnacle of his speech was the controversy about our ability to live without food. He claimed that Sungazing is a doorway to make this very possible and very real.

(Note: this is true, how I was able to go ninety days no food.)

Some locations feel different than others. Experiment. I found Sungazing in nature the most enjoyable with tranquil results. It is the road not the destination that needs to be addressed. Embrace the journey. Have an open mind and be receptive to notice change to occur.

He adds more to HRM's comments:

Every civilization has practiced Sungazing, it predates recorded history. It was used to cure disease, destroy harmful bacteria and generate vibrant health. Sunlight was used in solariums of ancient Rome, ceremonies by native American tribes. The Suns influence appears in Arabian culture, Hinduism, Buddhism, among the Druids of England, the Aztecs of Mexico and the Incas of Peru.

Hippocrates and Pythagoras wrote extensively on the use of Sunlight to gain optimal health. Greek physician Antyllus wrote much on Sun therapy, prevents an increase in bodyweight, and strengthens muscles and makes fat disappear. Reduces swelling as well as hydropic swelling.

In the earl 1900 hundreds sunlight was found to contain ultraviolet light which is detrimental to about every known, bacteria, that is Bad for our health. Anthrax, the plague, tuberculosis, cholera, staphylococcus, the colon bacillus and dysentery can all be destroyed with varying amounts of Sunlight.

The invention of penicillin in 1938 and other antibiotics to a large extent caused the with-drawl of Sun therapy.

The nerve ganglia in our body, particularly in our abdomen are similar to electric wires for receiving and conducting photons of light. This light energy is constantly being collected by the skin, the eyes and sent to our internal organs and cells. This process is called metabolism.

Skin health is an important component for proper absorption of Sunlight. The human body needs a balanced spectrum of light as part of our daily diet. Without it "cabin fever" a common term coined from lack of Sunlight that relates to depression, actual term, Mal-illumination syndrome for deficiency and the negative effects from lack of actual Sunlight and the replacement of natural light with artificial and harmful pink or cool white fluorescent light."

For example, just visit any nursing home or for that matter most assisted living facilities and look at all the bodies starving for more energy and vitality that Sunlight could improve.

Chapter 7

The Sungazing Journey begins

Phase 1: The Healing of the Mind

In an attempt to create a steady flow of information, I purposely am formatting this volume with fragments from my journals on sungazing, which contained 344 entries including additional data not related to the journals to prevent boredom and to make more interesting.

Therefore, I have decided to divide my journal information into the same three phases of the HRM Protocol—Phase 1, the first fifteen minutes gaze time, Phase 2 will be to thirty minutes gaze time, and Phase 3 to forty-five minutes. Following each section, I will give a brief summation to my experiences and how the experience has influenced me.

I will also include additional information of my research that creates a well-rounded understanding of sungazing from ancient sungazing cults methods, including how religions focused on the sun.

I also documented my gazes on Facebook most often with images taken at that time with comments about weather and my experiences. I am including many of these in order to create an intimate experience with you, the reader, so you can share the same visual sensory situations I felt at that moment.

My Journal Notes
Began Sungazing (Surya Yoga)

March 1, 2014 (ten seconds)

My first experience sungazing, I followed the procedures recommended in the HRM Protocol. I began staring at the sun naked-eyed in ten second increments. I found it very difficult to focus, kept squinting, and eyes watered like crazy. First time ten-second session was shared with Wendy at sunset on the docks at Salt Ponds Marina. Wendy experienced the same watery-eye symptoms herself.

(Note: *Also, on this day, I stopped wearing my prescription sunglasses, which I have worn for years due to sensitivity to light and poor vision, caused by a traumatic brain injury from electrical shock.*)

March 3, 2014 (twenty seconds)

A couple days later, I added another ten seconds of gazing time to the first ten seconds I experienced the gaze prior. I went to the neighborhood Buckroe beach just before sunrise. Facing east, I took off my shoes and socks and buried feet in the sand, fifteen to twenty minutes before sunrise. Once I had centered and grounded myself, I began with standing meditation posture (ji gong/qi gong). I watched the sunrise before I began timing with alarm of my total sungazing time.

Once I finished gazing, I turned with my back to the sun and placed the palms of my hands over my eyes. In Hatha yoga, this is known as palming. Also, I was performing a self-reiki method into my eyes at same time. I was amazed and enjoyed a number of colorful and dynamic images as I stood still until the sunspots disappeared. My eyes are already adjusting better to the Sun but still squinty and watery.

I went home immediately and drew the images I had just witnessed with crayons.

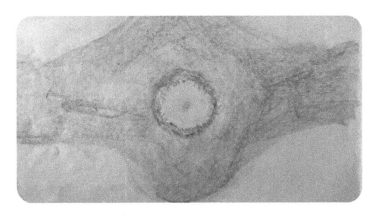

March 4, 2014 (thirty seconds)

The next day, I performed same routine, with sungazing total time still less than one minute. I came home again today and drew with crayons, the different colors and images today then yesterday, beautiful.

Also began walking on the beach. I'm feeling more energized and motivated, more so than in years since my "grand illumination," I like to call my electrical accident (LOL).

I returned to drinking my solar water again and varying sun teas, after taking time off during the winter months. The freezing cold temperatures were breaking all of my glass containers.

March 8, 2014 (one minute)

(Note: As I stated earlier, I will not be entering all of my journal entries to keep it interesting.)

A celebration is in order. I hit that magic first minute this morning. My eye complaints, in relation to being as uncomfortable looking at the sun, have subsided significantly. My eyes are still a little watery but improving every day.

Today I realized how much I enjoy sungazing to the extent that I am already addicted to sungazing.

(*Note: Amazing in such a brief period of time I am already seeing improvement in my eyesight. I am starting to have flashes of momentary good vision which occurs sporadically and is spontaneous.*)

March 13, 2014 (one minute thirty seconds)

Still at beach doing same ritual pre-sunrise and at sunrise, including my walks barefoot in the sand.

(*Note: I experienced an interesting phenomena I described as "an interior opening of my mind, feeling of an inner holographic experience. Felt as if I was present inside the cave of Brahman as an observer." I experienced residual effects of this experience as it lingered throughout the rest of the day.*)

Again, I drew images with crayon.

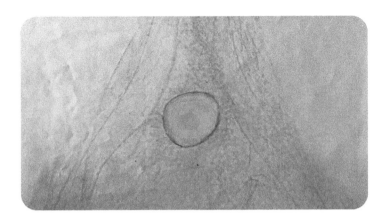

March 16, 2014 (one minute fifty seconds)

I had visions of double stars following sungazing today.

(*Note: I discovered a day or two later it was the seal of Solomon.*)

Drew the image with crayons.

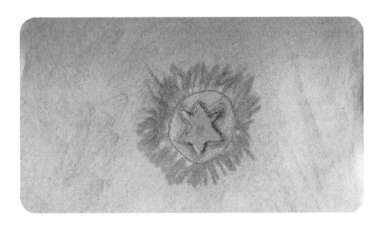

March 22, 2014

(*Note: I have noticed the last two or three times at sungazing, I have begun to physically feel an increase in my interior vibrations just moments before the sun crests the horizon. This morning was exceptionally strong. This occurs at the precise moment that the seagulls begin their wails and chirps of joy. As soon as the sun peeked above the horizon, the vibrations suddenly subsided. At last I have obtained the ability to feel the subtle but powerful intensity of the coming sun! Awesome! No doubt I have to thank the birds for teaching me how to recognize this physical phenomena so well. I am inclined to believe now, this is the reason roosters crow out loud in the morning. They can feel the telluric currents as the sun is rising!)*

March 27, 2014 (two minutes fifty seconds)

(Note: I have found myself becoming more and more obsessed with experiencing the sunrise every morning. I am so excited when I wake up in the morning that I cannot get out of bed fast enough to get to the beach and watch the sunrise.)

I set my alarm thirty minutes before sunrise each morning. This gives me time to get dressed, make a cup of coffee to go, and to walk to the beach.

As part of my routine, I've begun my sungazing from the same location on the beach, standing with my bare feet in the same spot. I'm working on creating an energy imprint.

I have also discovered that even when my alarm, which I set before I gaze, goes off for me to quit, I don't want to stop my gaze.

I feel as if my body has become magnetized; the sun is drawing me in toward it. I can feel the sun's positive attraction.

(Note: this is when I realized the similarity a plant experiences always being pulled in the direction of the sun.)

(Note: for the past several days, I have been experiencing a strong desire to help others. Two days ago, I hand-delivered a heartfelt letter I wrote to a neighbor, who had recently suffered a severe stroke, with my offers to help.)

My emotions have been raw with so many tears of profound joy and desire to help others, it has left me emotionally drained.

I had to take an afternoon nap, which is very unusual for me to do.

I'm so full of hope.

I drew with crayons again.

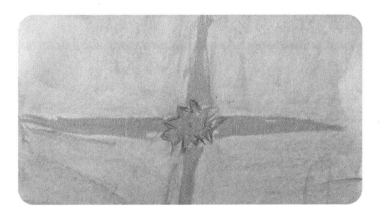

March 28, 2014 (three minutes)

(Note: For some reason, I could feel the energy this morning before sunrise. I was able to feel the same vibrations I have been feeling but for longer duration—and felt more subtle. I couldn't understand why today the vibrations that I typically feel were weaker. At that time, the only difference I could tell was a low-level haze on the waters horizon.)

As soon as the vibration stopped, I opened my eyes, and the sun was cresting the horizon.

I drew with crayons. Last drawing for a while. Who knows how long before I visually document once more?

(*Note: My eyesight keeps improving enough to notice, and I wonder if my cataracts are leaving.*)

My barefoot walks on the beach I consider my meditation and contemplation time, much like the Himalayan Forest monks in India that predate the Buddha, who walks in the woods of the wilderness. I do this exercise three to four times a week.

I have taken on a new route walking on the beach. I walk the majority of the time in the water of the breaking surf which is an indescribable experience itself.

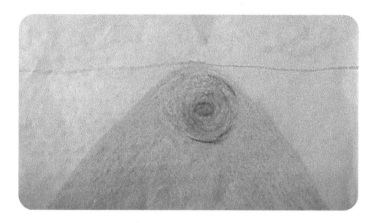

I estimate I am walking between three to four miles distance. It takes one hour and fifteen minutes.

If I live to be a thousand years old, there is one event I will never forget.

During one of my beach walks, a couple days later, the first of April, I was walking along the beach's edge headed toward the fishing pier that was my turn around point.

Instantly I had a premonition: I knew my mother was going to die on my birthday!

Immediately the tears burst from my eyes like projectiles. I literally saw them shoot out in front of me as I was walking.

Oddly enough, within seconds, I felt a calmness of peace consume me, and I was comfortable with the terrifying and very emotional information.

The entire experience was so surreal, in a moment's time, my emotions rocketed from the serenity of the seas shore to the death of my mother on my birthday, which is just over two weeks away.

I found myself speaking to God and saying, "If it's your will, it is okay with me."

A very peculiar comment for me to even consider saying. It was automatic, no cognitive thoughts or reasoning.

When I returned home from my walk, I couldn't wait to explain to my girlfriend the events that had just taken place. I said to her, "While I was walking on the beach today, I received a message my mom was going to die on my birthday on the nineteenth."

She grinned a big smile and began joking about the voices in my head, telling me I really was crazy because "there is nothing wrong with your mom, and her health is good. She's happy and content and doing well."

April 13, 2014 (five minutes ten seconds)

(*Note: Today I noticed that during my gaze time, I feel as if my body is becoming magnetized by the sun.*)

The sun's energy field is having such a powerful effect on me that I can literally and physically feel the sun's energy field pulling me forward toward the sun without any assistance from me whatsoever.

Awesome! Recently for a brief period, I have noticed that the bald area atop my head has become covered with a short, almost like baby fuzz over the entire bald spot. I am certain that my hair is starting to grow back. Awesome, awesome!

(*Note: my vision has surely improved significantly. In the morning when I wake up, my vision is perfectly clear. I can see Wendy lying next to me and appreciate her beauty without having to spoil the moment by trying to find my glasses. The lenses are typically dirty from the day before.*)

During the day, I have noticed there is a range of distance that I can see perfectly well. Hoping all ranges to improve to be able to see at all distances. I am very hopeful that I will experience continued improvement with all the varying distance ranges.

April 14, 2014 (five minutes twenty seconds)

Because I have gained the ability to recognize some different subtle energy vibrations, I have decided to be flexible enough in my experiment to maintain the integrity of the HRM Protocol and to create a more controlled environment to measure and document my personal experiences, which is what this book is all about. In other words, making this experiment my own.

Prior to my research on sungazing, I had researched and explored a plethora of information to aid me in understanding my newfound sensitivities since my "grand illumination."

(*Note: For some time, I had developed the ability to identify the earth's natural telluric fields. Today I started to use that skill and align myself with the north and south electromagnetic streams. These are the strongest energy streams on the planet and are the mechanics of a magnetic compass which tells us the direction for navigation. It is also the easiest for me feel consistently, and I do it without any aids or devices.)*

I want to remind everyone I am a trained yogi and reiki master, and I trained in the Japanese karate system of zen for years, so I have a familiarity with a number of ancient energy systems and cultures. I also have been a fan of bio-rhythms since the '70s.

I've also begun to include in my morning gazes on the beach a Kriya yoga meditation I learned from Paramahansa Yogananda, with eyes partially open, allowing light to enter, in combination with my already comfortable, (ji gong/qi gong) still meditation posture.

I have also added pranayama breathing, yogic breath, including the breath retention I learned from the study of kundalini yoga.

The inner vibrational feelings I have been recognizing have really become magnified in their intensity since doing so. I am not just feeling a subtle vibration as before. That was little more than a tingle in comparison to what I'm beginning to witness now.

(*Note: I can also feel the energy where my heel contacts my instep on my feet, particularly on my right foot. I feel as if I have electrical impulses transferring into the sand from my foot, like a static electricity.*)

This static condition only occurs when my bodyweight shifts forward due to the powerful pull of the sun's magnetic forces, placing more weight on my toes. I believe if I didn't make a mental effort to resist the powerful magnetic attraction of the sun, just to close my eyes and give into the sun's magnetic field, I believe I would tumble forward to the ground.

From my research, I have discovered this is not an uncommon occurrence to sungazers who practice the ancient art form long enough.

I also am convinced by research studies, which claim our body's blood hemoglobin (which is filled with iron) is reacting like in a plant where photosynthesis occurs. In a plant photo plasma is the blood (which is filled with magnesium), and I am being pulled toward the sun, exactly in the same manner as if I were a plant or tree that always turns itself or its leaves in the sun's direction.

Using another ancient kundalini yoga technique known as Khechari Mudra, I hold my tongue curled backwards with the tip of my tongue touching on the soft pallet of my throat. This sacred technique utilizes the tongue as a switch that connects the lower energy systems of the body to the soft palate, which is directly below the pineal gland. When I perform this Mudra, I can physically feel the tingling of energy moving from my tongue to the soft palate of my mouth. I can feel the temperature increase, and I flinch at the electricity stings.

April 16, 2014 (six minutes fifty seconds)

(Note: This morning was one of the most beautiful sunrises since I began to sungaze, and I took several photos to show Wendy. It was really a pleasant gaze this morning, and I feel so solemn. I cannot honestly express my emotions with the realization that my mom is dying soon.)

April 19, 2014

 Leo Walton   •••
Apr 19, 2014 at 3:37 PM · 👥

Hi all...been sometime since I visited fb and became engaged in its diversity... But in keeping with the spirit of the day I felt motivated by a number of folks to say thanks for all the birthday wishes and how great it feels to be 61...and to share the profoundness of this consecrated day...a day to believe in the power of our cosmic influences...my loving and generous mother experienced the end cycle of her human existence this morning at the precise moment of sunrise becoming magnetized by the polarity of the sun leading to her ascension into the light...my life to be changed for all time by this glorious and remarkable experience... I cannot imagine a better birthday gift...peace to you all and thanks

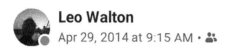

Leo Walton   •••
Apr 29, 2014 at 9:15 AM • 👥

Death...is it something to fear...as the soul of our universe (sun) rises in the east each morning ...and sets each evening in the west...the sun is not lost...the sun has not disappeared... the sun is only hidden behind the horizon... we do not fear...we know the sun will return to shine on us again...such is the human soul (sun)...

(Note: There was no sungazing today to celebrate on my sixty-first birthday. My mom transitioned peacefully at 6:32 a.m., precisely at sunrise this morning.)

Wendy felt horrible about the comments she made just a short time ago when I shared my premonition. She apologized many times the past couple days, and I told her it's okay, she was right. My mom was in good health, but she declined suddenly falling out of consciousness just a few days earlier.

I am a big fan of numbers, and I pay attention to their importance and symbolism.

If you take 04-19-14 as written, the numerology equals 1.

If you take the time of my mom's death at 6:32, the numerology is 11.

My address is 1st and 11.

This year currently as I do this edit, it is 10-10-19. She has been gone over five years, and I have discovered what a valuable gift she gave me for my birthday.

In the past, my birthday has always been about me. It's funny, I don't think of me anymore. When I think of my birth, I think of my mom. She was always a very generous person who loved to give things to people. She was my biggest fan, I miss her very much.

April 20, 2014 (seven minutes)

Yesterday was my birthday, and today is Easter. The fact my mom transited yesterday made this morning's sunrise on the beach a special moment today.

Wendy, who has never come to the beach to gaze with me in the past, wanted to come along for the celebration.

As we approached my well-charged energy spot to sungaze, I saw a fishing net buoy lying in the bull's eye of my energy grid. Now I can say in nineteen months of gazing from the beach, in that exact spot, there were never any gifts. What made the fishing float so significant for me and Wendy was how very strange the event was. For weeks, Wendy and I had been looking (unsuccessfully for weeks), scouring the beaches to collect some of these floats to decorate our new home, which we were hoping to buy in the mountains. We wanted to bring a bit of our life here to there. All I can say is, "Thanks, Mom."

April 22, 2014 (seven minutes twenty seconds)

Returned to my favorite spot on beach today. The inner vibrations I've been feeling just about the entire experiment have intensified to about the same as a continuous shiver.

(*Note: my body has now begun to vibrate with tremors with enough amplitude that my arms are quivering.*)

April 25, 2014 (seven minutes forty seconds)

(Note: My favorite spot on the beach is getting lots of use lately. Today the intensity of my interior vibrations were off the chart. After five minutes of gazing time, I could feel them coming on. I began to get that wavy feeling inside, like being drunk, and then the vibrations increased in strength to the point that my arms and hands were shaking significantly. It made me uncomfortable being there in a public location where someone could watch me.)

April 28, 2014

(Note: The weather not conducive for sungazing today. However, Wendy made a comment this evening I felt was important to document and share. She stated that recently she had noticed "a significant change in my demeanor." She continued saying that I was "calmer and less anxious as typical." My reply was that I felt calmer and more relaxed, not bothered by much. I am very happy to be where I am in life and in love with a beautiful woman who loves me to death. We were beginning to forge our life together unencumbered for the first time since we've been together, almost four years. We both agreed that it is because of the sungazing and in combination with my walks for the shift.)

May 1, 2014 (eight minutes fifteen seconds)

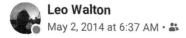

Leo Walton   •••
May 2, 2014 at 6:37 AM • 👥

Hi all...this year is my time to come out of the closet...so to speak... In 2007, I experienced an NDE from electrocution...suffering a TBI as one of the results... my recovery time has been lengthy and the numerous stages of emotional upheaval have been challengeing...sometimes more so for others then myself...since that time...I call re birth...I have exhibited a strong will to attempt to become a better human...I fell in love with Yoga and became a Yogi...I became most interested in bio energetics and became a Reiki Master...I was totally catapulted on a spiritual journey and I became an ordained minister...having hands on experience on a plethora of concepts...researched and with self testing...I am going to share my latest endeavors which I want to recommend to all...it will change your life in ways you cannot imagine... It is Sun Gazing...more to follow...

On the beach this morning, the sky was hazy and cloudy. I decided since I had walked over that way, I would spend a few minutes measuring energies anyway.

The air temperature is the best and warmest to date. It's sixty-seven degrees and the first time I'm not bundled up—comfortable and wearing a long-sleeve T-shirt.

(Note: I could still feel pre-rise sun energies, but it subdued again because of cloud cover. The ever-present slight pull toward the sun was still a part of the equation. I definitely have developed a magnetic connection with the sun to be able to feel it on an unfavorable a gazing day as today.)

This time, I didn't experience any of the typical sunspots or colors at completion of my gaze for an example, but my confident attitude and focused intent created some benefits from the time I spent gazing. I figured I may do a second gaze in the evening and spend some time with Wendy at sunset tonight.

(*Note: Having to spend a lot of time on the computer the past three days, I've been having to wear my close-up reading glasses to be able to read the screen. The prescription glasses of my last eye exam are definitely having a negative influence of my vision at other times when I'm not wearing the reading glasses.*)

May 3, 2014 (eight minutes fifty seconds)

(Note: *this is the only negative experience I suffered from sungazing, and it was as a direct result of gazing too long, too soon. I preset the timer, but the alarm failed to function on the new sungazing app, so my gaze time ended up being between twelve and thirteen minutes during the afternoon time. The sun was very intense today, and I was already tired from walk on beach earlier today.*)

I was so exhausted I could have just closed eyes and fallen to sleep while standing there. Even with intense sun conditions and being sleepy, I didn't have a good feel or connection with time, and the sun magnetized me to the point where I stared until alarm sounds. If Wendy hadn't been present, I probably would still be gazing.

Later in the evening, I encountered one hell of a headache that originated at the rear of my head in the location where the spine lays adjacent to the visual cortex. I am one who seldom has a headache other than my customary "brain spikes" from my temporal lobe epilepsy, which I have had on going since my electrocution (grand illumination) in 2007.

I am convinced the headache was from too long of an exposure to the intense afternoon sunlight. I do want to comment that the afternoon sun is not as gentle as the morning sun.

Understanding the pathway of sunlight as it enters the eyes, the sunlight goes through the retina to the optic nerve, which then transfers the light signal to the back of the brain where the hypothalamus resides. The hypothalamus is like a mirror, and it reflects the light it receives to its target, the pineal gland.

I wonder if the headache was a complaint from my medulla oblongata?

(*Note: Following that particular gaze, Wendy and I both experienced sunspots on most anything whose surface was white in color, and this lasted for some time afterwards. We also noticed that when marina lights were turned on, they had a more pinkish hue. Definitely gazed beyond our current capabilities and comfort zone.*)

May 4, 2014 (nine minutes)

The morning sun is my favorite time to gaze. Everything about it is calming, no pedestrian noise, and the sound of waves crashing on the shore. I can meditate without any significant distractions or interruptions.

Another attempt at using the new sungazing app, and the alarm failed for a second time. However, not wanting a repeat of yesterday, I set a backup alarm to prevent another headache.

I fired that app. It was removed from my cellphone. Be warned, my recommendation is to test them numerous times before your gaze if you use one.

May 13, 2014 (ten minutes forty seconds)

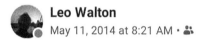

Leo Walton   •••
May 11, 2014 at 8:21 AM • 👥

It's Sunday again and my topic today is influenced by sun gazing...not to forget those great teachers of the past...the very first thing that God gave was light...the sun the reason for ALL life on earth...as human beings and all things we are a manifestation of this light...artist have always used halos of light in their paintings to represent holiness therefore we accept holiness as light...pure light that shines in spirit... An accepted law in all faiths is only what is pure can purify and what is holy can sanctify... Light then can sanctify because light is holy and light is the purest form of God's spirit...sun gazing is mans acceptance of this law and the joy of God's spirit...

I didn't catch the sun at sunrise this morning even though conditions were very good. Just decided to enjoy bed a few minutes longer for a change. When the sun came up, it was low on the horizon, thirty minutes after sunrise. Today the sun was very powerful and pretty intense.

(*Note: My eyes were pulsing like crazy, and I had to close them tight a few times and refocus, but good viewing.*)

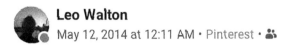

Leo Walton
May 12, 2014 at 12:11 AM • Pinterest • 👥

The Greeks called this sun blooming...I want to use this yoga asana at sun rise at buckroe beach...but Wendy said hamptonians have a different perspective...

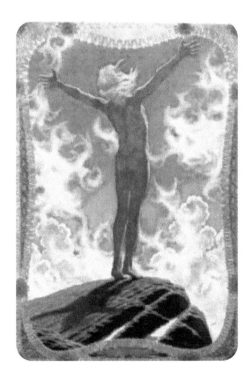

May 15, 2014 (thirteen minutes)

My gaze time increased this morning, a larger jump than typical or recommended. Had to chase the sun around a little today due to the cloud coverage, but my gazing time was actually a couple minutes longer than noted. The sun was at a good, comfortable intensity even though I had to wait longer to allow the sun to rise above clouds on the horizon. My alarm sounded for a while, but I didn't want to stop because the experience was so comfortable, and I was drawn in by the sun's magnetism. I could feel the attraction stronger today, more so than in a few times gazing. Again, the weather conditions had not been very accommodating. I have created a new set of guidelines to focus my intensions. Everything felt good, and I was not trying to rush. I was paying attention and listening to my body and responding accordingly. I would have no difficulty looking a lot longer at the sun, but the alarm had been sounding for minutes, and the sun had been hidden by the clouds.

When gazing, time seems to pass very quickly.

All good. Going to walk on beach today.

May 19, 2014 (fifteen minutes)

It was a beautiful sunrise this morning, and it was timed perfectly to coincide with the one month of my mom's passing on my birthday.

It was also my first milestone with this experiment, reaching the fifteen-minute duration of sungazing timeframe on HRM's Protocol and completing the first of his three-phase program.

My gazing in the morning began before the sun had risen and then continued until the sun was high enough on the horizon that the reflection of the sun began on the water near me. As the sun's altitude increased, that reflection ran across the bay and touched the Sun, making a connection of dedicated light current to me.

This is when I began to time my gazing time. If I timed the entire event, I'm assuming I most likely was gazing closer to twenty minutes. However, the time I gaze like this is wonderful, I don't want to stop. I could keep going. I know my body and can tell my limits. I feel because my kundalini is awake that it may be possible that my nervous system is already experienced and trained to be able to handle increments at a little faster interval, another experiment.

I've been holding my arms and hands up in differing positions, I think of a cormorant sunning his wings.

All right, it's time to provide the Summation of Phase 1. What an incredible journey this has been so far.

Chapter 8

Summation Phase 1:
The Healing of the Mind

HRM claims that the first phase of his protocol is the cycle of time necessary to allow for the healing of the mind. By completing this segment, one has satisfied the requirements necessary to be able to quiet the mind and control the emotions under any circumstances.

First, I have to state that the benefits I have gained following completion of phase 1 can only be identified as spectacular, miraculous, and wonderful!

Up until the time I began my first gaze, my life had been plagued with a number of chronic disabling maladies, due to an accidental traumatic brain injury caused by electric shock. It had been seven painful and frustrating years with great loss and suffering that I had endured before I did my first ten seconds of sungazing on March 1, 2014.

I prefer to call this life-changing event my "grand illumination."

Because of the damage to my optic nerve and vision center, my eyes became extremely sensitive to sunlight or any other bright light for that matter, so I had no choice but to wear sunglasses. All my prescription glasses, even the bifocals, became sunglasses, and I wore them constantly, day and night.

To complicate matters, my vision was deteriorating at a noticeable rate, and I was diagnosed with cataracts. Cataract growth is a common condition of those who survive electrocution by alternating current electricity.

During my research, before I started to sungaze, I learned that a number of people shared testimonies of improvements in their vision. Armed with this information, I decided to remove not only my sunglasses but all prescription lenses from use for the duration of the sungazing experiment. I felt this was the only way to monitor any significant changes I may encounter in my vision, whether it was improvement or further deterioration.

I did, however, use a pair of over-the counter reading glasses exclusively for reading, or you wouldn't be reading this today! For my eye health, now I do wear sunglasses when walking in the sand, driving long distances in the car in bright sunlight and when doing water sports such as kayaking.

Within a very short period of time, as I documented in my lab journal, I noticed improvement in my vision. I could see in the mornings when I first got up to begin my day, and I would experience moments during the day of clear vision at certain distances.

The biggest difficulty I had with vision was night blindness. I suffered so much from scattered light that for years, I made every effort to not have to be on the road when it was dark. It was so bad that I would become disoriented and not know where I was, and I missed lots of turns. So in order to protect myself and others on the highway, I avoided night driving.

Today I can get into my automobile and drive anywhere I want to go with confidence again. I can see clearly without interference whatsoever from traffic lights, automobile lights, or street signs. There is no longer anything that bothers my night vision.

The physical benefit overall is that my eyes are no longer light sensitive.

Another serious issue I had was a sleep disorder, which was severe enough, I was prescribed sleep medication for years. For me, sungazing recalibrated my circadian rhythm, and it helped heal my damaged pineal gland, making it stronger and more efficient in the manufacture of melatonin, which is the critical hormone necessary for sleep. It improved to such an extent that my personal physician removed me from my sleep medication.

(Note: Now that I am discussing medications, I want to let you know, I was on six different prescriptions when I began sungazing. In the nineteen months of my two experiments with sungazing, I was removed from most of the prescribed drugs, and within months of completing the experiments, I had been removed from all prescriptions. Today in October 2019, I have not been on any medication for almost five years, and I have not experienced any illness such as flu or colds in that time.)

It feels great to have returned to great health, and I am sixty-six years old.

I should have stated that I had two sleep disorders. The second one was night sweats. For seven years, I would perspire so heavily that some nights I would awaken as many as four times a night with my T-shirt soaked, and occasionally I would have to change my bed linens. None of the physicians I was examined by over the years—and again, there were forty—could really offer any diagnosis or any real suggestions to improve my night sweats. Of course, there was always "take this or take that," which did little to reduce the frequency.

I did a substantial amount of research on this topic, and by accident, I discovered that my some of my symptoms such as the night sweats ran parallel with what I had experienced at the time of my accident—a sudden kundalini awakening.

A brief explanation is when an individual's kundalini energy has been activated, their internal electrical voltage increases ten times the normal amount. To provide an example, the average human being produces about the same amount of electricity as a hundred-watt incandescent lightbulb. When the kundalini is activated, it flips a switch to produce thousand-watts of power.

In many of the eastern traditions, especially the Hindu and Buddhist, the invention of yoga was for one purpose. When yoga was created by the ancient sages, the intentions were to prepare the bodies bio-energy systems, including the nervous systems, the endocrine systems, and the lymphatic systems to be to handle the tenfold increase in voltage the human vessel would receive. Therefore, if a person has not been adequately prepared to handle this voltage, this person will become subject to many negative physical and neurological ailments, particularly mental and emotional stresses.

Today in America, it is estimated that as high as 30 percent of institutionalized mental patients are suffering symptoms associated with a sudden kundalini awakening because they are not prepared.

For me, the result is all good news here too. I no longer have night sweats, and I am able to sleep an entire night uninterrupted. I cannot express the difference it makes in your daily life to go seven years, without a full night's rest—full sleep. Today I sleep through the night more often than not. My mental condition is more peaceful, less agitated, and less prone to anger. I have more patience and get frustrated much less. This is a significant improvement from my pre-sungazing, and I am grateful for having completed this sungazing experiment.

Early in my recovery, as my brain was healing, I would experience flashes of intellect that I affectionately refer to as cognitive shifts. These cognitive shifts were frequent in the beginning, and the frequency of occurrence declined to the point of nonexistence.

I mention this because during the same time period I experienced the cognitive shifts, I experienced ice pick stabbing pains in my forehead and temples that would occur without warning. No matter what I was doing, I would instantly become 100 percent debilitated and nonfunctional from the pain. Luckily the pains were hard and fast, and the pain didn't linger. It was the mental anguish afterwards that lasted; it would really take the wind out of my sails for hours the rest of the day.

I learned I had symptoms associated with temporal lobe epilepsy, and I was prescribed medication for people who have epileptic seizures. It was an odd experience because the ice pick pains moved around to different parts of my head. One time, the ice pick would pierce my temple on the left side. The next time, it would be the right, and sometimes I would feel the stab in the middle of my forehead.

I often wondered if it was some kind of brain warfare going on—brain battles between the two hemispheres for either right brain or left brain for dominance and control.

By the time I finished the first phase of the HRM Protocol, I was 100 percent free of any ice pick stabbing, along with the debilitation and suffering.

When you damage your pituitary gland, which creates your brain chemical serotonin, and the pineal gland, which manufactures the brain chemical melatonin, together, these two are responsible for our mental equilibrium. The correct amounts keep us within a certain range of emotional stability. Therefore, I have been on two prescriptions as hormone replacement therapy to replace the chemicals my brain didn't manufacture properly since 2007.

Being conscientious in my research, I scheduled an appointment with my psychiatrist. During this visit, I was able to easily convince my physician to reduce the dosage of the medications. She did so graciously, reducing the dosage by 50 percent.

I was elated.

One common ailment found with people who experience a TBI is that they suffer from chronic fatigue syndrome, which I call lazy man's disease. I say this humorously now, when really, it's no laughing matter. It is a very serious condition where the energy to be motivated is absent and is replaced by fatigue and lack of desire. At this juncture in my sungazing, my typical daily energy levels and stamina have improved measurably. I don't seem to be suffering from chronic fatigue as often.

I have had a lifelong condition of suffering from sinusitis and allergies. I have been surprised by significant improvements a benefit I didn't expect but am happy to receive. Springtime is usually a miserable time of year for me. With all the pollen, I used to eat sinus tablets, Claritin and Sudafed, like they were candy. I still have some symptoms, but they are not severe enough to warrant taking any medication. One great improvement has been my sense of smell. I notice all types of smells and odors now that I never paid attention to in the past. The spectrum of smells has really increased. Some of the foul ones are much stronger, which I could have done without.

A week ago, I pulled a quadricep muscle in my right leg, I heard the muscle tissue snap as the fibers tore. I had slipped while walking barefoot on a grassy hill. Having experienced this same type of injury once before, years earlier, I was familiar with the severity of the injury and the debilitating affect it has on your daily routine. The immediate intense pain was enough that it made me nauseous for minutes afterwards. Not only was my leg extremely sensitive to localized touch, but I could physically see the bunching of the torn muscle tissue sagging in a clump above my knee cap.

Seriously, within twenty-four hours, I was walking perfectly. I was amazed at how speedy and short duration my recovery time. I still was experiencing localized pain at the site of the muscle tear, but I felt my healing time was miraculous to say the least.

My mental condition is more peaceful, less agitated, and difficult to anger. I have more patience and get frustrated much less—a significant improvement from pre-sungazing.

Emotionally, I do feel that being calmer has allowed me to experience more joy and love in my daily life. I'm more caring and considerate of others and have a passionate desire to share my phenomenal success and convince as many people as I possibly can into at least trying sungazing.

Another injury related to TBI for me was I began to cuss—not just an occasional curse word but about every other word. This was Tourette's Syndrome, and the more excited I became, the more filthy my mouth produced a language that was very unbecoming, and I had a stuttering problem. I cannot tell you how horrible it is to realize the things that came out of my mouth. It was very embarrassing and really a detriment to my confidence and made me withdraw from any type of social life.

This improved immensely but didn't end.

The hair on top of my head four months ago was void of hair except for a few straggly hairs in the very front, but it has now begun to grow. Not just a few, but my entire bald area is covered with new hair growth with is unbelievable. At this time, I expect that my hair is going to return.

In 1994, I was in a serious automobile accident, and it seriously injured my back. I have suffered from a herniated disc between L#4 and L#5 which causes extreme sciatica that I have been having spinal injections for pain since. The relief I get from pain typically lasts an average of four months. Incredibly, I haven't seen any significant discomfort since the last injection on the first of February, and I am due now for another scheduled injection. Even though I am at the end of that four-month timeframe as I complete Phase 1, I am not experiencing any of the typical symptoms that flare up as the cortisone injection wears off.

I hope this continues as I progress through the other two phases of the HRM Protocol.

I have been walking on dry sand now for a couple weeks although very sporadically. Much harder than walking on the wet sand or even in the surf. After doing it a couple times, I can feel a significant increase in the energies being that they are sustained longer into the evening. I was walking about four miles which is taking an hour and half. Because of hot sand and crowded beaches and HRM's suggestion of forty-five-minute timeframe, I decided to decrease my time accordingly and do between forty-five minutes and one hour.

For a while I have noticed the refraction of light colors pulsing from the sun. I am experiencing the entire light spectrum. Recently I have been able to notice that the energy leaving the sun is in a spiral and it is traveling toward earth with a counterclockwise direction, opposite of what is thought considering the sun's protons are positive. Because if we were on the sun, they would be leaving clockwise, but our perspective is receiving the energy; therefore, the energy is reflected like in a mirror and are opposite. I believe the same is true for the earth energies, and if an object is above our atmospheres like the international space station, they will be perceived by the astronauts, for example, leaving the planet with a clockwise rotation, which explains why plants, flowers, and seashells have clockwise rotation, while the construction of a spider's web is being influenced by the sun and has a counterclockwise rotation.

(Note: *At this time, I cannot say enough good things about sungazing. I love it, it has been one of the greatest experiences of my life. The healing I've received—there are no words to express.*)

I also am determined to reduce the strength of my blood pressure medicine. I plan to schedule an appointment with my primary physician in near future. I believe in strict professional engagement with many doctors for all my extreme experiments.

I believe it is possible for my herniated disc to improve dramatically and possibly heal my other aches and pains are improved and less frequent. I'm still having brain spikes but not as often and for less duration, which is okay with me.

I'm hoping by the time you read this page and my testimonial on concluding Phase 1 of my sungazing experiment that you have an understanding of my passion for this ancient art of Surya yoga, known today as sungazing. Already the significant improvements in my life have been nothing short of miraculous. In a short period of four months' time, I've experienced the elimination of pain, the elimination and reduction of dosages of medications, the improvements in my vision, gained the ability to sleep the entire night, enjoying peaceful undisturbed rest, and my emotional state is euphoric.

Okay, I have completed the long list of positive improvements that I have benefitted by sungazing.

Now I would like to address some comments about sungazing being the key to unlocking the so-called dormant parts of the brain. I want to discuss the extra sensory gifts I have experienced.

I'm very excited about the combination of sungazing and walking barefoot on the beach. I am a believer that the two together are from dealing with sun energy and earth energy, the yin/yang.

I have experienced a number of clairvoyance events. First, I want to remind everyone about the events surrounding my mother's death, the vision I had of her passing more than two weeks before my birthday.

This ability is known as clairvoyance or precognition and is the exhibiting the ability to perceive events in the future beyond normal sensory contact.

I will continue this conversation at the Summation of Phase 2, thirty minutes of gaze duration time.

CHAPTER 9

PHASE 2
THE HEALING OF THE BODY

 Leo Walton
May 17, 2014 at 7:15 AM · 👥   •••

Getting out of bed earlier every day to catch that first
ray...requires reason...here's two...
13 min 20 sec

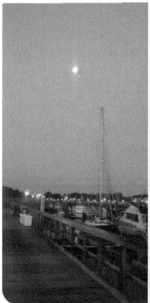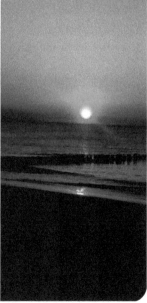

May 20, 2014 (fifteen minutes ten seconds)

This morning was fifty-eight degrees Fahrenheit, about the same as yesterday. Gotten a little cooler, I have only been able to wear shorts and take my shirt off once. It won't be much longer now till I'll be back to my Bohemian attire.

As typical for this time of year, the weather allowed me to piggyback days of gazing in the morning together. I have noticed when I am able to accomplish, I can feel the sun's vibrational energies. I feel as if I'm one of the sun-powered toys I purchased for my mom. It has a small solar panel on the pedestal and is a dancing scarecrow like in the farmer's fields. This morning as I stood with my arms outstretched just below being parallel to the surface of the earth, my palms facing toward the sun, my left arm began to vibrate. After a minute or two, the vibration became more like a shaking—a pulse-like movement of my entire arm, not violently, just subtle. Within a few minutes, my right arm began joined in doing the same vibrating, increasing into a shaking on its own. In a short period of time, both arms became synchronistic and began to shake with the same resonance. This shaking reminded me of a tuning fork or better yet two tuning forks that became joined in harmonic sympathy.

When both my arms began to pulse and shake in rhythm, the sun generated energy, felt natural, and was not uncomfortable.

The experience was actually very interesting, and without actually monitoring the exact time, I believe it probably began at eleven or twelve minutes into my gaze.

Maybe now that the weather is getting more consistent and I can get a number of days gazing in sequence, I'll be able to experiment and observe this phenomena. Also, my gaze times are getting longer, allowing more opportunity for this type of event to occur. I feel a strong connection to the sun now, and I know the sun feels it too, I believe I am developing a relationship with the sun, as impossible as that sounds. That is the way it presents itself to me.

I have totally relinquished myself to the sun with 100 percent confidence that it has my best interest in mind.

I have absolutely no fear from it at all. All my doubts and hesitations have been replaced with love for it.

May 24, 2014 (fifteen minutes twenty seconds)

It's been a few days since the sun made its availability at morning or afternoon. Sunrise this morning was beautiful, gold, gold color. Pleasant temperatures at sixty-one degrees Fahrenheit, no humidity, with a pleasant light breeze.

The sun's vibrations are becoming increasingly easier to tap into, which makes me ecstatically happy. I was concerned that having a few days off I wouldn't be affected as much as the last gazing. Again today, I'd say twelve minutes or so, my arms start to tremor and bounce, today was a little different. The last time my left arm started first and then right arm began to do the same thirty seconds or so later. Today both arms started at the same time. I was holding my arms higher in different positions seems a little more comfortable for longer duration. Everything in little steps for big rewards.

I could feel energy moving early, mostly on the left side of my body, being able to feel and locate the north-south electromagnetic stream has become simple to achieve, not experiencing any difficulty. Seems like I have a more difficult time with the subtle energies, when wind is blowing, I think it is because the wind activates other senses in the body and brain causing an interference of sorts.

I'm still watching the sunrise, probably at least three minutes before I start the timer.

Soon I imagine I will have to change that habit as my gaze duration lengthens. A lot has to do with atmospheric conditions and haze and cloud cover, etc.

Today is my mom's wake at the Assisted Living Home where she died—a very good way to start the day.

May 25, 2014 (fifteen minutes thirty seconds)

Wendy and I did sungazing together today at sunset. We decided to experience gazing from the marina docks. We began sitting lotus style on one of the floating piers, but after a few short minutes, Wendy says, "Let's dangle our feet in the water." I'm glad we did, it was a very pleasant experience. we had our feet submerged about halfway up our shins.

Once I had acclimated to the water and returned to gazing, I completely lost all recognition of my legs, absolutely no feelings whatsoever. It was a very surreal experience. The sensations, or lack of, makes me want to try again, this time in waist or chest high water, as some of the Eastern Jain Indians do.

Wendy commented afterwards that "she noticed when we first began gazing with our legs in the water, that the water conditions were slightly disturbed from the east wind and then noticed a calm area form close to us at the dock we sitting on." She had stopped gazing before me because I have increased my time a little more than she; therefore, she was able to observe the environment more closely. She said, "The calm water physically extended at a distance of seven to eight feet from us and the dock itself."

She was curious if the energy of the sun passing through us into the water was the cause. I don't know, we will monitor more closely next time. Good observation Wendy.

One thing I learned was the reflective glare being this close to water at sunset is terrible and distracting. I had to hold my hands up entire gaze time just to block intense sunrays, which are much more penetrating and hotter than the rays directly from the sun alone. It was a powerful learning experience.

Note: HRM is a Sheetambar Jain, pronounced Swe-tambara in Sanskrit. This cult's yoga has six essential practices which include six lying or standing asanas. The standing posture which I have been doing automatically that I related to qi gong is very similar in the Jain tradition and is called Kayotsarga, pronounced Kaussaga. Their philosophy is relinquishing any bodily activity. Most of the tirthankaras of Jainism are depicted in this standing posture. It means to give up one's physical comfort and body movements, thus staying steady while standing or lying and concentrating on the true nature of the soul.

May 27, 2014 (fifteen minutes fifty seconds)

A beautiful sunrise but hazy conditions—had to stop clock once. This is distracting to vibrational and magnetism with the sun, but it is what it is. Tomorrow is another day.

Happy with progress, the ninety-day mark is approaching quickly.

May 28, 2014 (sixteen minutes)

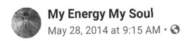

My Energy My Soul
May 28, 2014 at 9:15 AM · 🌐

A perfect 'Good morning' ~

My Energy My Soul

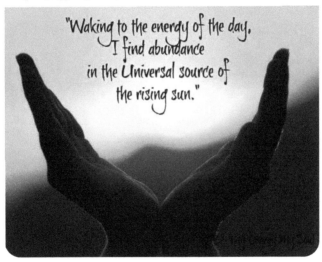

"Waking to the energy of the day, I find abundance in the Universal source of the rising sun."

I was a little late getting to the beach this morning. It was thirty minutes past Sunrise, and it ended up being an intense sungaze event. Wasn't hazy, it was more humidity then haze. I spent maybe as much as half of gaze time on my tip-toes. I can feel the attraction of the sun and believe there is a balance position while on my toes that corresponds with the north/south field and in combination with the sun's magnetism similar to the image of the "Greek" method for sungazing.

I'm beginning to get more comfortable with my arms raised. Seemed to help my balance while on my toes. I will experiment further.

(Note: I watched a one-hour YouTube lecture by HRM, and he said to "hold your arms like a greeting, elbows bent about ninety degrees with your hands up and pointed toward the sun." He also said to "get the most energy walking, to do it in dry sand." I didn't have any arm tremors today; however, I could feel pulsing, intensity of sun, and doing other postures made time seem a little slow today. Still doing breath retention but haven't made it a routine procedure yet. Still experimenting, just hit-and-miss, random trials.)

May 30, 2014 (sixteen minutes ten seconds)

Following a couple days of unfavorable conditions for sungazing, I experienced good integration today. I was a little later getting going, didn't catch the exact moment of the sunrise. The sun is always a little more intense on my eyes if I'm late getting to the beach because from just awakening, my eyes are still used to darkness, so rushing to adjust so quickly to the brightness is stressful to the optic systems. When I'm early and catch the sunrise, it allows my eyes an opportunity to a slower more comfortable pace, making the experience pleasant. Also, we have to take into account my gaze time is getting longer, and the sun becomes more intense the higher it gets in the sky.

June 1, 2014 (sixteen minutes twenty seconds)

This is the anniversary date of ninety days sungazing.

Great way to celebrate with a beautiful sunrise. I experimented again standing on my toes and holding my arms in different positions. No vibrations today but great energy. The early stages of Phase 2 of the HRM Protocol is going well. I am so excited to be able to do this experiment.

I do feel a lot calmer and have more joy and love in my daily life. I'm more caring and considerate and have a strong desire to convince people to investigate sungazing themselves. I'm putting it out there with my morning photos of the sunrise with accompanying encouragements. I love it.

June 2, 2014 (sixteen minutes thirty seconds)

Absolutely gorgeous this morning. It was a little cool at fifty-one degrees Fahrenheit, but with no wind, I did have to wear a fleece long-sleeved shirt.

(Note: I didn't try to do anything method-wise, I just relaxed and gazed at the sun, my arms slightly extended. The vibrations began as was typical in the past, and this morning, the vibrations entered and filled my torso. This is a first-time experience. As a

matter of fact, I could feel the vibrations beginning to sneak down to my thighs.)

(Note: HRM suggests just relaxing and do nothing physical. Think I will try to do this approach for a bit of time longer before experimenting with the Greek method further/ I find it's good to change things slightly to be able to measure the differences in energies.)

June 3, 2014 (sixteen minutes forty seconds)

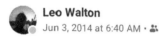

Leo Walton
Jun 3, 2014 at 6:40 AM · 👥

Morning all...sun is shinning bright today...Sungazing... 16 min 40 sec...can feel the healing energy flowing through my core...

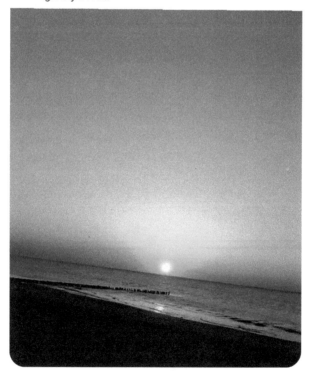

I arrived a few minutes just after sunrise today, and I went right to sungazing. I was in the relaxed posture, no breathing exercises, no experiments, just totally becalmed and available to feel the experience. I was amazed at how fast time went by. I was lost in another world. It was a magnificent meditation. I could feel the vibrations inside my entire body; they were subtle except in my arms. I experienced some physical tremors but felt them decreasing in intensity. I believe the reason is because the sun's energy is now spreading throughout my entire body.

Amazing, simply amazing.

June 4, 2014 (sixteen minutes fifty seconds)

Another spectacular and beautiful sunrise. The sunrises sometimes reason enough to rise out of bed and walk the nearly three-quarters mile to the beach in itself. I have set new record of sunshine, which allowed me to sungaze for five consecutive days.

A pod of dolphins swam a short distance offshore—always a wonderful experience to witness and share. I just relaxed and enjoyed it all. I feel so lucky.

June 5, 2014 (seventeen minutes)

Another minute down the pike. Today I watched at sunset from the decks of my floating abode, the Sea Spirit. It was an intense experience; I wasn't barefoot and grounded to earth or water, and the power and intensity of the sun at sunset is much harsher on the eyes to me. The gradual energies as the sunrises allow your eyes to adjust more calmly rather than *bam* in the afternoon. The sun is at its most powerful when you begin and gets weaker as it sets.

(*Note: the Egyptians would gaze at sunrise and sunset, and I can tell you the energies have a different effect on your systems. I'm just learning this myself, and it is too early for me to offer reasons, but I will as I mature.*)

Another magnificent milestone today is my first grandson was born, and I celebrate seven beautiful grandchildren.

June 6, 2014 (seventeen minutes ten seconds)

This morning was fabulous. I just relaxed and was—*I am*. I just let the energy flow. I can still feel when it gets to flowing into my core. It is the greatest experience, the most wonderful drug—hypnotic. The time passes so quickly, I don't want to stop.

How can this be? I am loving it so much, I never want to stop!

I am so addicted!

Fired up about helping a young man in his thirties with ALS and another friend's daughter also in her thirties who suffers from a brain cancer. Both have families with multiple young children.

(*Note: received four e-mails from Hira in response to my request to represent his methods of sungazing here in the west. I'm so excited. His personal e-mail which had referenced to ALS was a powerful documentation and encouragement to spread the word about sungazing. He sent me a number of contacts articles and a book written about him by Vina Palmer, MBA,* Living on Sunlight, *which I have already referenced as the guide to follow to safe sungazing.)*

June 7, 2014 (seventeen minutes twenty seconds)

What can I say? A great morning for sungazing—the temperature in the middle sixties Fahrenheit. I managed to catch the sunrise on a ninety-second video for the first time since I began gazing. The routine vibrations are incredible. Time just goes by so quickly, I actually catch myself going, "Damn it" when the alarm sounds.

I received info from ALS guy yesterday about his research of damage to the eyes from looking at the sun, that he obtained from Wikipedia. Not a good way to start a trusting relationship—I didn't get a very positive vibe from his message.

I had contact from the ALS guy's closest friend today, the man who hooked me up with him, this morning about his friend. I requested his friend's info to forward to Hira personally. No response as of yet. I don't believe he is interested.

I have done some deep meditation on this and wonder if it's too late for him to be a candidate. Maybe he has already accepted the fact that he is going to die and doesn't want to put his friends and family through any more suffering.

It has to be very sad for everyone.

I have learned that it is common for those chronically ill, especially those with a death sentence such as ALS, and that it is what I have determined it to be—a death sentence. The current mindset today of all medical professionals is to give up. There is no hope, get your affairs in order, you're a dead SOB, period. So sad.

There needs to be one individual that says, "I want to live and try sungazing" with a positive attitude, someone that is brave and has not given up. It will happen when the time is right, and it's meant to happen.

If my book saves just one life, heals just one person who suffers, it has served the reason I wrote it.

June 9, 2014 (seventeen minutes thirty seconds)

 Leo Walton   •••
Jun 9, 2014 at 6:59 AM • 👥

Morning all...clouds on the horizon...trying new things...video and photo...Sungazing 17 min 30 sec...have a great day...

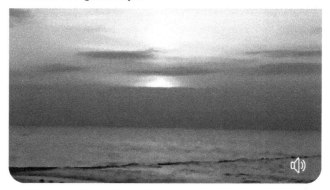

I had to wait for the sun to get high enough to clear low-lying cloud cover this morning. However, it turned out to be worth the wait. It was a good gazing experience. Again I just relaxed and allowed the energy flow to flow through me like a river. It was fabulous.

(Note: Sungazed ten days in a row—new personal record. It really makes a difference overall

with being able to sungaze every day, if possible. It is worth the effort if the weather is favorable.)

June 12, 2014

Since the last entry, I have been to beach two times—once on the tenth, and it was too much cloud cover. The second time on the eleventh, and I could have gazed, but was there was no wind, and the insects were horrible. Between the no-see-ums and mosquitos, they carried me away before the sun ever rose.

It was just too difficult to deal with the torment to have a quality experience. The conditions haven't been favorable in the evenings either.

Also, this morning, it was a slight drizzle with foggy conditions. Been raining off and on all day. Looks like a wash today.

June 13, 2014 (seventeen minutes forty seconds)

It was a lot of cloud cover this morning left over from last night's thunderstorms. While it was difficult gazing this morning because of low-lying clouds traveling north covering the sun, being a start-and-stop kind of day, it took forty-five minutes to get the allotted time in today. Again, the bugs, the no see-ums, still out with no wind this morning. Definitely an aggravation, and I will have to look into using a natural bug repellant on this type of day.

Heard from ALS guy last night requesting information be sent on Facebook which I couldn't get info from e-mail to Facebook. I looked up other options and located the book

Living on Sunlight on another free e-book site and forwarded it.

I have my fingers crossed.

June 14, 2014 (seventeen minutes fifty seconds)

Not my most intense experience. There were heavy clouds on the horizon at sunrise, remnants from last night's storms. Was a stop-and-go gazing with sometimes obscure sun.

(Note: When I performed the palming method at the end, I noticed an oval diamond-shaped blue image surrounded by the gold of the sunspots. The color is light blue like sky blue. I feel this is the infamous spiritual and mystical blue pearl spoken of in Vedic text, sometimes in other philosophies called the blue diamond or pyramid.)

June 15, 2014 (eighteen minutes)

Finally, a good gazing experience. I switched back to qi gong posture for this one, and I noticed a lot more vibrations in my hands and arms. I can definitely feel the energies more with my hands to my side and turned out toward the sun. The blue diamond is getting sharper and clearer in form.

June 16, 2014 (eighteen minutes ten seconds)

 Leo Walton
Jun 16, 2014 at 7:15 AM · 👥

Morning all...beautiful sunrise...Sungazing 18 min 10 sec...

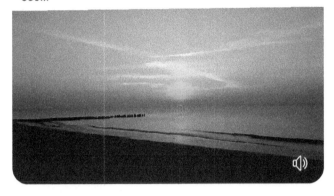

 Leo Walton
Jun 18, 2014 at 6:48 AM · 👥

Morning all...yesterday reached 100 with feel of 120...another hot one today...humid on the horizon...another beautiful day as summer solstice slide in...Sungazing 18 min 30 sec...for those who are avid experienced meditators...the blue diamond has begun appearing just before 18 min Sungazing time while palming afterwards...awesome...just awesome...

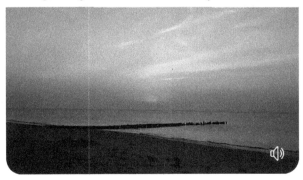

Another good sungazing experience. The vibrations are beginning sooner and lasting longer. Blue diamond.

June 17, 2014 (eighteen minutes twenty seconds)

Yet another fantastic experience today. The vibrations are lasting longer and longer. I am surprised and happy about this. The blue diamond is ever present now at the end.

June 18, 2014 (eighteen minutes thirty seconds)

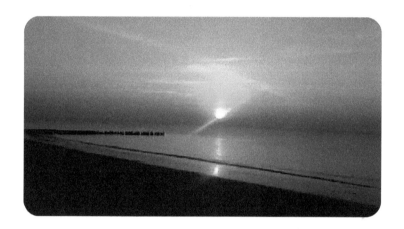

A great gaze today. The vibrations started after a short time, the earliest to date, and lasted almost the entire gaze session. There was a little intermission here and there, like an ebb and flow, but for the most part, the vibrations were pretty constant. I have determined the vibrations are really evident in my wrist and hands, since changing posture to qi gong again, with my wrist resting on my hip bones. This posture seems to accentuate the vibes. Time will tell. Just awesome gaze. The blue diamond, pearl, pyramid—all the similar shapes appeared.

June 23, 2014 (eighteen minutes forty seconds)

It is hard to believe it has been five days since I gazed on the nineteenth. It was a good day, but I have been hard pressed to get out of bed lately. I have been really tired past couple days, the temperatures have risen during the day to a hundred degrees Fahrenheit, and I have been working hard in it, preparing everything for the kids to come home for summer. Decided I needed to rest longer.

The twentieth through twenty-second weren't very good conditions anyway—rainy and cloudy. Even the evening sunsets haven't been favorable for sungazing. Yesterday on the twenty-second, I even went to the beach amidst heavy cloud cover and high winds. No luck but made a cool video of the storm front over the water.

Today my alarm didn't sound, so was a little late getting to beach, but it was a great gaze. The vibrations started early into time and seemed to level out closer to end of the gaze. However, I noticed when the vibes slowed, I could feel an unfamiliar pulsing in the core of my body that was synchronized with my hands and arms.

I also had a slight image of the blue pearl centered in a cross pattern of green.

June 24, 2014 (eighteen minutes fifty seconds)

Today's temperature was sixty-eight degrees Fahrenheit. A nice breeze was blowing out of the east south east. I wore long sleeves and sweat-pants, but it was a beautiful sunrise this morning.

My mindset was difficult this morning. It was encumbered with too many people and commotion on the beach. The warmer temps are bringing people to the beach, a lot of them walking their dogs. It takes me a little time to get used to the loss of peace and quiet, so it did have an effect on me today. I need to work on being able to focus better by being able to go inside.

I captured some nice images and video of the sunrise.

The vibrations didn't seem to mind the distractions, they started early again and are lasting a long time. The pulsing resonance is becoming customary.

I did yoga yesterday and today, and when I'm meditating and calm, I can feel the same pulsing as if I were sungazing. It feels good and maternal—reminds me of a mother's heartbeat when you are a baby.

We went to Busch Gardens on Sunday, had a great time, and had an experience. There was a man and a woman with an adolescent teen girl who was crippled, wearing headgear, and confined to a wheelchair. They were waiting at the exit gate to get her on the merry-go-round for a ride. When I noticed the folks, for some reason, I got goosebumps, and I could feel my energy strengthen.

I observed the lack of any empathy from the hordes of people standing in line and just watched these two parents struggle to get this paralyzed girl onto the ride. Even the employees of the park were absent in assistance.

I mentioned it to Wendy, and as we slowly walked away, we were discussing my opportunity to help this little girl and her parents. Anyway, I ended up going over and offering to help. This man was so fast and experienced I wasn't much help and barely made contact with the girl. The people were so grateful for someone to offer to help instead of ignoring them. Even after this, my goosebumps rose.

June 25, 2014 (nineteen minutes)

Today I gazed at sunset time, not my favorite, but had a good gaze till last few minutes. The clouds began to obscure and block the sun. I didn't experience the typical energies.

Doing yoga now consistently, and I am noticing a significant energy connection between my thumb and middle finger when meditating. This is called the Ida Mudra and is known as the gesture of the Lunar Nadi for balancing the lunar channel of energy.

It is a calming, cooling energy method that reduces blood pressure and stress, relaxing the body and breath. I can feel the pounding of my heartbeat resonating to the point that my entire body begins to vibrate. It's awesome, its same frequency I experience when sungazing.

Also, I have noticed that following sungazing, the blue image I see palming is becoming softer and more and more pearl shaped, but still is angular in form sometimes.

June 29, 2014 (nineteen minutes twenty seconds)

Was a great sunrise today—captured a nice video, had seventy-two degrees Fahrenheit temperature, light winds from the east which are off the ocean, and a beautiful sky.

I performed the Surya Mudra for a while. This Mudra is called the gesture of the sun for activating the fire element. It enhances radiant energy in the mind and body. It increases metabolism and clarifying our life purpose. I decided after several minutes, it is best used for static meditation, not something as dynamic as sungazing.

Also did yoga, meditation, and a sunbath for my spine.

Love starting my day this way.

July 4, 2014 (twenty minutes) milestone

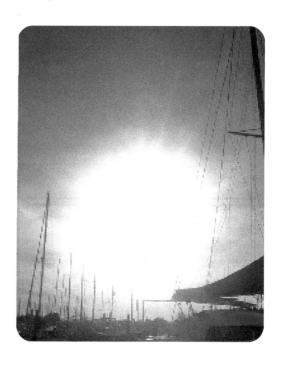

Who would guess a few months ago that I would reach the ability to physically stare at the sun naked-eyed for the duration of twenty minutes? My sungazing on the fourth of July holiday was aboard the Sea Spirit and at sunset, before the annual fireworks display. It was a good gaze.

July 5, 2014 (twenty minutes ten seconds)

Everyone's gone today from the Marina. There was a large crowd down enjoying their boats for the holiday.

(Note: I began to gaze at 6:00 p.m. It was a bit too soon to start, and I could feel the intensity of the sun's heat on my eyeballs. I also had a torrent of energy enter my optic center, making my pineal gland ache when I was attempting to focus my gaze using the HRM posture. I did the exercise on the top helm deck of the Sea Spirit at sunset.)

Since I was a little early, I gazed intermittently for brief periods, and then I would wait twenty to thirty minutes taking a break. I could tell a significant difference in intensity of the sun, with a thirty-minute time difference as it got closer to Sunset. I am beginning to recognize that the longer you continue to sungaze, the duration gets longer, and the sun's intensity increases in several ways. The intensity, heat, the pulse frequency vibration, and the speed of the sun's spiral rotations increase.

July 6, 2014 (twenty minutes twenty seconds)

Another great morning. I arrived at the beach just as the sun was cresting the horizon, and it appeared as a big yellow-gold globe of fire.

Good gaze—the temperatures nice and cool with consistent breeze. I could tell that I had been away from grounding, and it felt good to reset. I have noticed I have been a little tense lately because I'm a little off my routine, but I'll fix that.

I had energies pretty early on. They didn't last till the end of my gaze but for a good while.

July 8, 2014 (twenty minutes forty seconds)

 Leo Walton •••
Jul 12, 2014 at 6:40 AM · 👥

Morning all...Sungazing 21 min 10 sec...I've noticed over the past week and a half that my appetite is less...hunger pains are lessening...they are farther between...I've dropped to two meals a day...did you know Sungazing and sun bathing are a natural cure for obesity...something special today...supermoon setting while sun is rising...

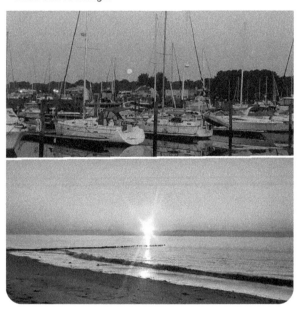

Once again, another great sunrise. It was a good gaze.

(Note: For the past couple weeks, I have noticed a significant decrease in my hunger pangs and loss of appetite. Not wanting to consume near the normal amount of food, I have gradually slipped into eating just two meals a day now. According to the HRM Protocol, this experience of not wanting to eat is little sooner than I expected to experience, but he lists the urge to stop eating most often begins after thirty-plus minutes gaze time duration. It is obvious that everything that is stated in the program has occurred early for me so far.)

July 22, 2014 (twenty-two minutes fifty seconds)

This morning at the beach, the clouds were on the horizon blocking the sunrise, so after three minutes, I returned to the Sea Spirit, finishing my gaze time from there after the sun arose above the cloud cover. It was a good gaze, and I am becoming more comfortable with the vibrational energies I keep experimenting and playing around with some Hand Mudras still.

(Note: I now have developed the capability to connect to the frequency of the sun's energy. The energies I've been experiencing are becoming routine and manageable.)

(Note: It is amazing now, and when I mention to others, they find it unbelievable, but if I place my middle fingers and thumb together either in Surya Mudra or Ida Mudra, within moments the energy begins to pulse and vibrate through my entire body. I have measured it and timed the frequency to be ninety beats or pulses per minute. In relationship to

the musical scale, it equates in the range of the key of C.)

I have had a long relationship with exploring the use of binaural brainwave entrainments, and most recently my interest has been in the 528 Hz frequencies.

528 Hz is considered a Theta brainwave state and affectionately called the love frequency, as it is scientifically associated with DNA repair.

Since I'm only eating two meals a day, I have shifted my mealtimes which breakfast used to be around 10:00 a.m. and is currently now a brunch at 12:30 p.m. or sometimes even later. Then the typical times for the dinner meal or sometimes just a fruit snack. One thing is certain: the quantity of food has dropped significantly.

My weight while doing a physical and blood work at my physician's yesterday was 186 pounds with all my clothes on.

I seem to be holding some fluid in my ankles as a symptomatic result of my blood pressure prescription that I am discussing with my doctor to reduce.

I was pleased with her response to reduce the dosage by 50 percent, but she insisted I take a water pill for a short period to reduce the swelling I was experiencing.

(Note: As my gaze time gets longer duration, the significant changes I notice as a result are slower and less frequent as my body and systems are attuning to the frequency of the sun; therefore to encourage flow in reading, I will be only commenting the future journal reports as the need to share pertinent information.)

September 23, 2014 (twenty-seven minutes fifty seconds)

 Leo Walton
Aug 8, 2014 at 8:48 AM · 👥

Morning all...yayyy...Sungazing 24 min 30 sec...been
tough to see the sun...pics

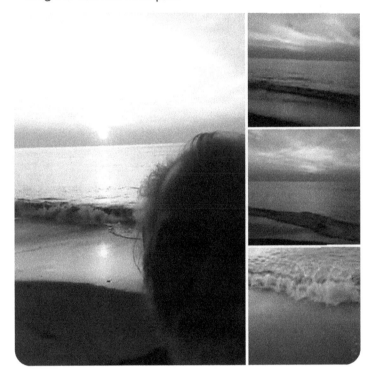

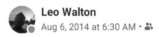

Leo Walton
Aug 6, 2014 at 6:30 AM · 👥

Morning all...Sungazing is tough when the sun is repeatedly obscured...walked to the beach with high hopes...didn't leave the hardtop...not dismayed but anxious for the sunset...yesterday...24 min 10 sec...another pic

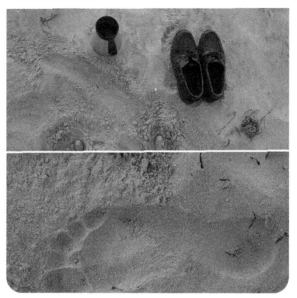

It has been exactly two months' time since my last entry, adding five minutes to my gaze time duration.

Wow, many changes have taken place since last entry. Summer has come and gone. The kids visited and have returned to their father's residence also.

Since April, I have lost four blood relatives including my mother and a cousin who I grew up together with and was more like a brother. I was closer to him in many ways as an older sibling.

The last of my dad's family, his sister who raised him as a baby, was ninety-two.

Wendy brought it to my attention that I am now the oldest living male on both of my parent's family sides—the patriarch, the alpha male.

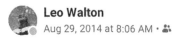

Leo Walton •••
Aug 29, 2014 at 8:06 AM · 👥

Morning all...Sungazing only 10 min...hopefully sunset will be clear to complete...

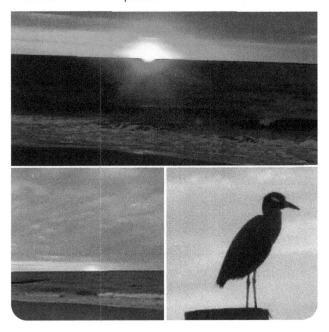

October 10, 2014 (thirty minutes)

I've come to yet another milestone—the completion of Phase 2 of the HRM Protocol for sungazing, the healing of the body.

Thinking about my start on this quest that began on March 1, 2014. That's over seven months of aggressive sungazing.

Under perfect circumstances, with the weather accommodating and the desire to rise earlier than the sun, walk to beach or wherever your location will be to gaze yourself. Fight off the biting insects, the sometimes cold, and many times requiring a second gaze in the setting sun to get your allotted time in.

To complete in the protocol timeframe of nine months would require all these things listed above to be pretty close to perfect.

I have to admit again I prefer to gaze in the morning.

Over time, I've been observant of my environment and have begun to notice some things that all aren't about the effects that sungazing has had on my person.

It's amazing really what I've taken in.

Sometimes I have been going to Buckroe Beach, which lies at the lower end of the Chesapeake Bay in Hampton, Virginia. It faces eastward looking out to the Atlantic Ocean.

From my vantage point and once I ground myself, barefoot in the sand, I allow my torso to relax, knees slightly bent facing eastward.

Closing my eyes, controlling my breathing, I tune in to the north/south polarity of the electromagnetic field that runs horizontal with the curvature of the earth.

Once I can physically feel the field:

(Note: the bandwidth associated with the north/south poles is extremely narrow and requires incremental movements in degrees just like with a magnetic compass; however, it has a U-shaped energy pattern almost like a house rain gutter. It's actually humorous when I think about it. The energy field pattern is shaped almost identical to the shape of a manmade magnet, the ones that you see in cartoons that look like horseshoes.)

Okay, I'm grounded, facing east across the Chesapeake Bays seventeen-mile fetch straight across the Atlantic, looking at Europe. I become light in the field, feeling like I'm floating in water within the close confines of the energy stream with my eyes closed, hands and arms hanging relaxed and loosely to my sides with fingers and palms facing toward each other, also within the north/south energy field.

Once centered and transfixed in a relaxed posture while standing, I mentally connect to my sensory systems and then tune my natural senses to attune my sensitivity range.

Doing this, I can physically feel an assortment of frequencies and vibrations. Some of these are the typical—feel of the wind blowing through your hair kind of stuff, but that's not what I'm referring too.

Yes, I notice the sensations minutes before the sunrises. Many changes occur.

I've become more aware of my surroundings and am noticing patterns associated with the solar wind that precedes the sun. It's called the bow wake of the sun.

I have also noticed a shift, a significant shift in awareness.

Leo Walton added 9 new photos.

Oct 7, 2014 at 7:38 AM ·

Morning all...only 3 min Sungazing this morning...64
temp light SW breeze...magnificent sky caught myself
racing to capture the brilliance 30 min before sun
rise...pics...all yeah run into some trouble yesterday on
the beach...

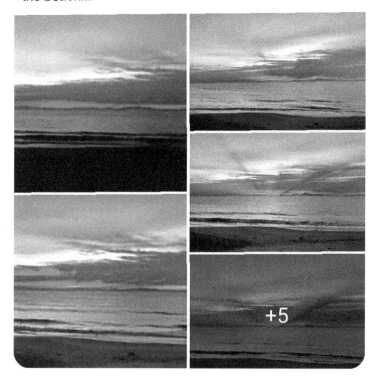

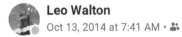

Leo Walton
Oct 13, 2014 at 7:41 AM · 👥

Morning all...no gazing this morning...yesterday captured Whitey snacking and this morning cats watching Helen standing on Sea Spirits swim platform...I love nature...it has been a living dream afloat on 4 different vessels for almost 20 years...soon I will be grounded to Terra Ferma...dirt...Forrest...mountains...and new wild friends I cannot wait to meet...pics

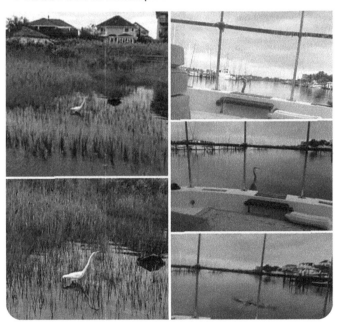

CHAPTER 10

SUMMATION PHASE 2: THE HEALING OF THE BODY

Thirty minutes gazing time—it is amazing at the amount of hair I have grown on top of my head. I don't look bald anymore. Balding maybe, but definitely not bald.

My vision has been inconsistent. I can see good first thing in the morning, but it quickly degrades soon after rising from bed. I notice when I use my reading glasses for extended periods, my vision worsens. I have started wearing two different glasses now. My vision driving was not acceptable.

I'm currently using over-the-counter glasses, 1.75 for driving and reading 3.25.

Also, overall, I would say at this time my vision is worse than it was at the Summation of Phase 1. Let me explain. I have cataracts on both eyes, but my left eye has significantly less vision than a brief time ago. I have noticed in past weeks that now when I look at artificial light, I do not see a single beam anymore, I see a larger diameter glow made up of many separate beams. In my opinion, it could be because the cataracts are becoming increasingly harder in texture, I don't know. Sometimes I can feel the cataracts on my eyelid, mostly from my left eye and many mornings I wake, and I have an abundance of this granulated debris in my eye I mentioned in last summation, similar to winkers but really crusty.

I plan on doing another visit soon with an optometrist.

The herniated disc in my back caused me much misery, pain, and lengthy periods of downtime, not allowing me to be able to go longer than four months without a spinal injection. I would literally become miserable and decapacitated. My last visit was February 10, 2014. That's seven and a half months, almost double the time between injections. I haven't had any of the typical symptoms, and I feel that I won't be getting anymore, at least for a long time.

My diet has been very good—lots of raw vegetables, bean burritos, etc., lesser amounts of dairy products, eggs barely. The biggest difference is that my hunger has continued to decrease. My last entry I was eating two meals a day. Currently I eat one meal a day, except for extraordinary circumstances. Social activities and traveling throws my routine off.

My hunger pains are less, almost non-existent. It's the empty belly and cravings that has been the most difficult to deal with.

Still drinking solar water, not much tea lately, but starting to want it again.

What is the most amazing is I have learned to tap into the frequency of the sun that provides fuel for our bodies. There is no question that my overall energy levels are greater than in a long time.

My body weight today is 175 pounds naked. I really don't believe I've lost but a couple pounds since I was checked by the doctor at 186 pounds with clothes, shoes, and pockets full in June.

I do know when I'm walking regularly, I do tend to lose more body fat.

My barefoot walks on the beach which began in the water and for about four miles long, started in March. Took time off while kids visited, however, the past eight walks have been in the dry hot sand, and I have only gone thirty minutes the longest. It's amazing, but I can feel an increase in my energy levels. I realize walking in itself is energizing, but this is immediate and long lasting.

I do notice this: the days that I walk, I become hungry a measurable amount. My exercise is burning more calories, and I feel I have not discovered the balance of energy for the increase in demand. As I walk more regularly, I will experiment with the energy levels and hunger. Both are good indicators of progress.

HRM states that you can give up food and eating when you can go three days without hunger pains, and homeostasis has been reached.

Wendy and I have done one serious detox several months ago, and we are past due for another. We also want to begin a once a week fast as routine. At present, we go twenty-four hours between meals which is considered a mini fast. I think we should go two days but drink plenty of healthy liquids once a week. We will do so as soon as we can get our routine synchronized with our plan to buying a house and relocating.

My mental state has been put to a very difficult test, and I have passed. Yesterday my scheduled appointment with my psychiatrist went in a positive direction. I'm doing so well that she reduced by 50 percent one of my prescription drugs. I'm really excited about this, I've been proactive with two doctors who are helping me reduce my medications looking for a new baseline.

Over the past several months, I have eliminated all prescription sleeping aids. Sungazing has reset my circadian rhythm, and I don't have difficulty sleeping anymore.

My blood pressure medicine has been reduced by 50 percent. However, for a while, I was beginning to have swollen feet and ankles, and the doctor said my BP script and my pain medicine both could have caused the swelling. She gave me a water pill temporarily till I adjust to the dose.

I don't have any swelling anymore. I think it is the blood pressure medicine. I have been on the pain medicine longer then I want to admit.

So soon the water pill will stop. My immediate goal is to try and reduce my pain medicine in half.

I feel good, fit, and strong. Over past several weeks, I've had four people I know who haven't seen me in a while comment on how good I look. Good for the ego and gives community support for adopting a healthy lifestyle including sungazing.

I also believe I have experienced clairtaction, which is the ability to sense being touched by a spiritual being—in this case, the spirit of a recently deceased person.

Chapter 11

Phase 3: Healing of Spirit, Soul, Achieving Homeostasis, Enlightenment, and Solar Nutrition

October 14, 2014 (thirty minutes thirty seconds)

Leo Walton
Oct 14, 2014 at 9:39 AM ·

Morning all...Sungazing 30 min 10 sec...I've begun the third and final phase of my personal experimentation with this most ancient and lost method known as Surya Yoga by the eastern Indians..at this stage in my research the growing list of emotional and physical improvements have been miraculous...currently my fellow sungazers number 8 and one is an optometrist... The list will continue to grow and grow...because the benefits are so huge that those looking to be healed...those looking for improvement in every facet of their life...will begin to see...hear others who have been so lucky...that they too will want to enjoy healing that is free...its safe...its a method and its simple...pics...

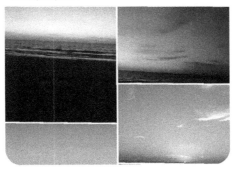

Another perfect morning sungaze experience at the beach, but the phenomena I experienced was paranormal.

I had a personal visit from my deceased mother, who has been dead now almost exactly six months.

She did not appear visually, it was an energetic encounter. I could feel her presence in the room. My hair stood up on my arms like it does when you rub a balloon against your skin, creating a static charge.

I verbally spoke to her out loud, but I didn't hear any audible sounds enter my ears, I could hear her internally answer my questions.

I know many will read this and think me insane, and then others will read and have experienced this phenomena themselves and have consolation that these experiences do happen.

The first time I experienced was in the time period of my NDE, in 2007, and it was with Jesus, whom at the time I believed in.

I encountered him in a white, cold environment—reminded me of a mental institute in the high security rooms. There was no color, no paintings, or photos or decorations, totally void of anything loose and not fastened down. There was no furniture with fabrics, only wooden benches anchored to the floor.

The only color that stood out in the surreal environment was the color of our hair including our beards and the penetrating blue of our eyes. We both have same color eyes.

Jesus walked into the room as I stood there, wondering where I was and why. He immediately sat down, and it was obvious to me he was suffering from great depression and sorrow. He sat down in his typical attire I had been taught to believe—a white pullover robe, much like a dress today in the United States or indigenous regions. The robe was tattered and was a faded, yellowed, and soiled cloth, Jesus sat down almost immediately and nervously placed his elbows on his knees and rested his bearded chin upon his hands.

His face was as white as a cadaver, with deep ridges gashed into his flesh, immersed beneath like trenches that contained ancient tombs filled with sorrows.

He just started talking out loud. He never engaged me and made any attempt to face me directly, he just looked down at the floor with a sad gaze.

He said, "I'm so tired of being this Jesus. All the years I have suffered because of the untruths and the stories being taught in my name that I had nothing to do with."

He continued saying, "He gets crucified every day and his existence is horrible."

I felt really sorry for the guy. It affected me so much emotionally that I passionately spent a year after my healing attempting to write a new bible and it took me a year to learn to read again and my first project was to write a new bible of truth.

I took the existing ones and was determined to create a better, more truthful version with positive techniques to reach a high level of spiritual realization.

After a year, I had only gathered enough truths from the Bible and positive tools to write a pamphlet. I became as discouraged as the Jesus I saw and ended my obsession because I realized in anguish at my failure, it was an impossible task.

It was then I realized why Jesus suffered. The bible had nothing to do with him, it was a story by Paul who was born eighty years after Jesus and was a murderer.

I was convinced that Christianity had nothing to do with Jesus. It was misnamed on purpose because in truth, the religion should have been titled Paulism or Paulanity.

Paul being a murderer would write such a horrible tale of violence, perversion, and create a blood cult that practices the rituals of devouring human flesh, drinking human blood, and torturous murders. That was his life, why he was in prison.

If Jesus had been accurately quoted and written about, it would be a positive, enlightening guide—lessons with tools to obtain illumination.

But instead, the current text is to create division, bigotry, hate, perversion, and merciless warriors that will kill in masses, men, women, and children.

The second time, in 2010, it happened, only this time with my deceased father, who died on Halloween, thirty-nine years prior.

If you are interested in numerology and synchronistic events, my meeting with my dad was thirty-nine years after his death, which occurred on Halloween in 1971.

The conversation was much like our last when I was eighteen. It was father to son, adult to child in nature.

It was three years following my "grand illumination," and he appeared one evening when I was playing my guitar. He was concerned for me, seeing my current physical, emotional, and economic status at the time.

The third time it occurred in 2012 was much different, being a USCG merchant marine boat captain and spending years afloat, living aboard my vessels for years. My current vessel is named the Sea Spirit. I experienced a paranormal event that had physical engagement with spirits in a unique way. Maybe it even could be called a possession. It was bizarre, a very unusual experience.

Following my "grand illumination," I became interested in yoga for physical therapy. I had not been able to turn my head to the left for two years, a result of the 220-voltage running through the nerves in my body and brain.

I joined a local YMCA and signed up for the yoga classes for the physical therapy benefits from it.

I didn't realize at first when I joined how profound the influence of yoga would play in my life.

It was wonderful for me. Everything about it was beneficial for me. In a short period of time, I gained full range of motion in my neck, and it helped strengthen my weakened left side while developing flexibility and provided a positive influence on my damaged confidence.

Another component was the general attitudes of the people taking yoga. They all were interested in peace, joy, love, and healing. My yogi instructor was no exception; she was a major influence in my participation. She encouraged me to further my quick passion for yoga and to enroll in a two hundred-hour, year-long training program to become a certified yogi myself to teach.

Over time, we became casual friends, and we both learned some facets of our personal lives.

It was interesting that we had some synchronistic things in common.

In brief, she and her husband were also into boating and owned a sailboat, and it was at the Marina I used to be in my sailboat, on the other side of the harbor my boat was in. Not only that common interest, but their boat was in my old slip that was just across from me now, and I had kept my other vessel there for about six years.

I also learned she had a son about twenty-four years old who was into motorcycle racing, a very dangerous sport.

Overtime, I completed my yoga training, becoming certified, and I stopped attending the YMCA classes, having continued my education with a second year of study training to become a reiki master.

During that time, I was Facebook friends with several people in my yoga circle, and I maintained frequent communication with all.

Suddenly, tragedy struck my yogi instructor's family, and her son was in an accident while racing his motorcycle. He was seriously injured and in a coma from head injuries. His mom, my yogi, had made several post on Facebook to keep her friends abreast of his condition as she stayed by his side for several days.

I'll never forget: she had made a late afternoon update about his condition and was concerned about his status. I carried on about my day, retiring to bed, resting peacefully, and awakening early, pre-sunrise the next morning as is customary for me.

I brewed my first cup of coffee and sat down to enjoy the hot cup of Joe, and within a few minutes, I heard this loud banging of someone's sail halyard clanging against the aluminum mast very aggressively. This is not unusual in very windy conditions and is more the norm being surrounded by sailboats; however, what really caught my attention was the fact the wind was becalmed, and it was the only boat clanging.

As the sun was about to rise and the darkness began to fade into light, I was standing at my back door, trying to focus on the vessel making all this noise, curious as to what the hell was going on, and wondering if it was a drunken sailor who had lost his mind.

The discovery was so shocking, it affected me like getting run over by a bus.

My entire being was overcome with emotions and energies that were so powerful, I was catapulted to react.

The sailboat halyard was on my yogi's vessel, and suddenly it stopped its violent rampage against the serenity of the harbor. Once I had recognized it, gaining a confident identification of the vessel, the harbor immediately returned to a peaceful and tranquil, dead silence.

I knew immediately my yogi's son was dead—the realization penetrated my being to the core.

This was confirmed a few hours later, on Facebook, by his mom's announcement of his passing during the night.

I was devastated and heartbroken for her and her family. I became filled with grief and was consumed with this powerful certainty that I had to go to her son's wake to express my condolences.

The announcement was made to the arrangements and location for the ceremony.

I traveled the forty-five minutes to the community church for the services and was pleased to see the wonderful turnout as the local community had embraced this family in such a warm and caring way.

I arrived and found a group of my yoga friends together, waiting in line to offer condolences to the father and mother of their deceased son. I had not seen them in some time.

It was a wonderful long line, and I observed the interactions between the two mourning parents, humbly and graciously accepting the generous heartfelt empathy and love of the community.

When it was my turn, I shook the dad's hand and expressed my condolences at this loss and turned to my yogi standing near him to give her a warm hug and to express my sorrow for her loss.

As I wrapped my arms around her and said I was so sorry, she immediately became agitated and aggressively pushed herself away from me, her emotions out of control, bursting into tears and disturbed, that I was concerned she was going to collapse to the floor. Her husband, seeing this, came to her aid, while I felt an overwhelming uneasiness to the point of paranoia. A numbness filled me, and I made a quick exit and left.

I cannot explain my feelings of this circumstance at the time, and it took me sometime to have an inkling of understanding as to what may have occurred, as crazy as it sounds.

My explanation is as bizarre as the events.

I believe in my heart that the son's spirit had intentionally visited his father's sailboat one last time before transiting to that other realm we all return to when our time on earth is final. I also feel his spirit wanted to communicate with me directly and to be able to use my living physical body to embrace his mother one last time.

As extraordinary and crazy as it sounds, I feel it can be the only reason based on the circumstances themselves.

The fourth time was in 2014 when I knew my mother was going to die on my birthday three weeks later.

The fifth time was the day after my mom's death on Easter Sunday with the crab pot float lying in my sungazing location.

Now six months later, the sixth incident I mentioned on this date.

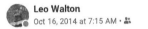

Leo Walton
Oct 16, 2014 at 7:15 AM · 👥

Morning all...sticky this morning...weather guessers said clear sky's but as typical they missed a little...walked to beach...heavy clouds east...I feel for Bermuda...I sailed there the first time in 1997...was a three week long adventure...was invited to the American embassy for July 4...wow the US does a superb job of celebrating ...best cookout ever...my next sail trip in 2005 was in a race...cruising rally...we finished 4th...but I couldnt beleive the mess Isabel caused a few years earlier...no Sungazing...pics...I always laugh at this sign...pics

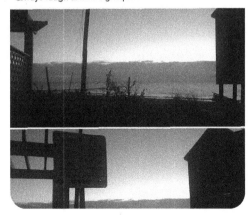

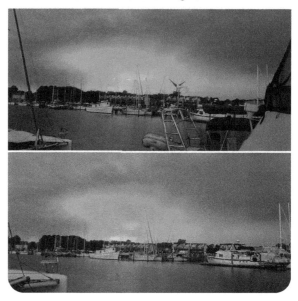

Leo Walton
Oct 16, 2014 at 6:36 PM · ·

Well no Sungazing this afternoon...but it was OK...check this sunset...10 mins ago...

October 20, 2014 (thirty minutes fifty seconds)

A pleasant gaze this morning. My mind and heart are excited because today I'm getting married.

October 24, 2014 (thirty-one minutes twenty seconds)

This morning, the temperature was in the low fifties, a little warmer because the wind was out of the west and on my back. However, the opposing winds and seas created a rhythmic pounding on the sandy beach of the shore that the sound created a vibration I could feel like thunder.

November 3, 2014 (thirty-two minutes forty seconds)

This morning's sungaze was a significant day for a couple reasons—one is the cold temperatures are upon us, *brrr*, and I have been relating my energy relationships to a new zero-point gravity theory.

Now that my sungazing times on the beach have gotten longer, I have become cognizant of many changes in the winds, the wave action of the sea, the influence of the north/south electromagnetic stream, and the magnetic attraction of the sun. I'm also aware of the resonant vibrational frequencies and how they affect me physically and mentally.

I intend to start purchasing some equipment to begin collecting data to compile a systematic approach to see how it all relates.

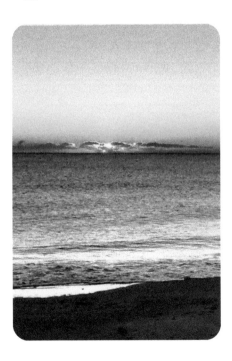

November 8, 2014 (thirty-three minutes ten seconds)

This morning's gaze at the beach, the temperature was thirty-eight degrees Fahrenheit. Being barefoot in the sand for almost an hours' time is beginning to be very uncomfortable and bone-cold. It takes me two hours to get warm afterwards.

November 13, 2014 (thirty minutes twenty seconds)

This morning, the sungazing event was cold again. It's becoming difficult to enjoy the experience when your bare feet become so cold, they become numb and stiff.

I have decided to make a pair of earthing shoes—earthing moccasins, I call them.

November 15, 2014 (thirty-three minutes forty seconds)

This morning gaze is the longest to date and was a typical gaze, however, I want to share how my eye exam went with optometrist on the thirteenth.

The doctor did the standard testing and at my request paid particular attention to my cataracts on both eyes. He actually took the time to take pencil and paper and draw them. He called it mapping of the cataracts.

(Note: He was in agreement with the other two prior optometrists I have had examinations with, that my cataracts were severe enough that he also recommended lens replacement surgery. That makes three eye professionals whose expert opinion is for me to proceed to have both lenses replaced on my eyes.)

Another inspection and evaluation he made was of a pair of sunglasses I have been experimenting for sungazing in glary conditions that are harmful to the eyes, like the salt water.

Over the last several months, these sunglasses have evolved beginning from a pizza box with holes to peer through and is currently in its sixth generation design that I have been using successfully for some time, and my satisfaction has led me to seek an expert opinion.

He was shocked at the function. He tested them by wearing to take his standard eye chart reading exam and claimed that he could see the chart significantly better than his own prescription glasses.

He was flabbergasted and excited enough that he insisted I apply for a US patent on the design.

His measurements of the alterations I made to a quality pair of Oakley sunglasses was that my apertures and their alignments were perfect size and placement.

He couldn't believe they measured so accurately with his specialized equipment and tools.

November 28, 2014 (thirty-four minutes fifty seconds)

(Note: This morning the sun was covered by cloud cover, and I did gaze for some time but wasn't feeling the energies as typical. I decided to go outside the normal safe time period in the afternoon as an experiment to finish my time because weather was declining. I began aboard the Sea Spirit about 2:30 p.m. The sun was too intense still, even though UV rating was at that time below 2.0—safe for skin not for eyes. I made several breaks for brief periods to wet my eyes and let my eye surface temperatures cool down. I do not recommend doing this. It is obvious that the heat and UV is harmful.)

December 1, 2014 (thirty-five minutes twenty seconds)

Finally, back on the beach for sunrise gazing, the temperature is fifty-four degrees Fahrenheit, and today was the first real test for my new earthing moccasins.

December 16, 2014 (thirty-seven minutes ten seconds)

 Leo Walton •••
Dec 12, 2014 at 8:10 AM •

Morning all...sungazing 36 min 20 sec...just short update...weather has been less then favorable all year for gazing...but particularly lately...

My gazing time has shifted since the sun has declined...I start after 2 pm now...

Miss those warm bare feet in the sand sunrises...lol

Think I'll buy an Island in the Caribbean... With white sandy beaches to spend my winters...
Pic...just now from the decks of the Sea spirit...

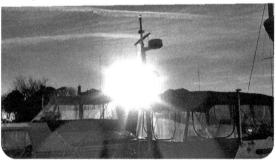

Since my last entry, I have for the most part been gazing in the afternoons aboard the Sea Spirit with the temperatures and conditions unfavorable in the mornings. However, now with having experienced the differences in energy measurements and frequencies between grounded and ungrounded gazes, I have come to some conclusions.

(Note: I've learned that I became both irritable and excitable from sungazing ungrounded at the beach compared to being ungrounded aboard the Sea Spirit. Big difference, and I feel it's because when grounded, the sun's energies flow through the body, energizing your systems and then passing to ground. Without being grounded, I believe the energy becomes stored more in the body, and the body becomes overstimulated, hyper, and sensitive. I do not think anything but short and occasional gazes would be tolerable ungrounded. HRM is 100 percent correct on being barefoot on earth. I wanted to experiment to find out why, now I understand.)

December 12, 2014 (thirty-six minutes twenty seconds)

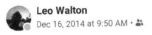

Leo Walton
Dec 16, 2014 at 9:50 AM · 👥

Morning all...Sungazing 37 min 10 sec...took advantage of warmer temps and calm winds...just returned from the beach... finally grounded...sun rise was missed but see pics...

Short update—since the sun has moved south so much because winter is near, I'm now gazing regularly after 2:00 p.m. The sun has lost a lot of its power. Think about it, the leaves fall off the trees for a reason.

December 17, 2014 (thirty-seven minutes twenty seconds)

(Note: I was running late for my morning gaze today. Didn't make it to the beach till well after sunrise at about 9:45 a.m. It is nice to return to back to the beach again. Lots of energy vibrations I don't experience unless grounded. I had a surge of Shakti this morning, which is the Hindu name given to the

kundalini energy. It was the first time I experienced kundalini this way, and it was a cold surge up my spine and was interesting with the warmth of the sun. A very powerful day, perfect weather, and my internal heat built up fast, so I stripped off my hat, coat, and sweater. My new glasses are performing great, and my earth shoes I made out of a pair of leather shoes, including leather soles. I simply took a large screw driver and hammer and removed the rubber heels so the shoes are now flat. I feel since they are natural products, I get the grounding effects without the freezing of my feet, and my energies make me feel like a rag doll, with an effortless stance. The energy flows are tremendous, overwhelming at times. I experimented at home with a copper bowl filled with quartz and a radio antenna. They seem to act as an amplifier of the energies. I use the bowl in my left hand and antenna as a pointer in my right. I can locate the north/south field as easy as a compass, and it is heavy with power. It creates a real heavy feeling with a tugging attraction.)

(Note: I am convinced using this makeshift device, I have found the narrow bandwidth of pole energy, the north/south electromagnetic field, sufficient enough that I have visually mapped the energy field with the antenna pointer. It also appears to be three inches or a little more in width. I will develop a more accurate measurement over time.)

December 18, 2014 (thirty-seven minutes thirty seconds)

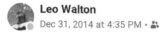

Leo Walton
Dec 31, 2014 at 4:35 PM ·

Hi all...happy new year...last of 2014...great day...Sungazing 38 minutes...afternoon sun...here's a great shot for the last sunset in ...14...from inside the helm...

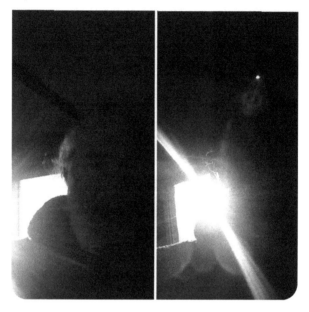

Another tardy appearance at the beach for my morning gaze, this time at 9:30 a.m.

The sun was white, bright, and a little intense at times. The air temperature was warm as well as the sun but not overpowering. It was a good gaze.

My body quivers were not as significant as yesterday, and I haven't measured the time into my sungazing when it occurs but believe it is still about the same as when they first began or when I first noticed—at about fifteen minutes?

The new grounding shoes are performing well. I cannot feel the ground as sensitively as barefoot, but I feel connected to earth, and my feet are comfortable.

(Note: An interesting observation is I have noticed about midway or a little further into my gaze, my attraction to the sun makes me lean into it. I also experience that when I close my eyes to lubricate them from being affixed and open so long, I immediately feel a disconnect from the sun's magnetic pull, and my body physically settles back into its normal standing posture and static balance.)

December 31, 2014 (thirty-right minutes)

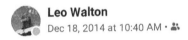

Leo Walton
Dec 18, 2014 at 10:40 AM ·

Morning all...Sungazing 37 min 30 sec...

Clear sunny and cool...wind north across water...brrr

See pics...one is from last night...sailboat...

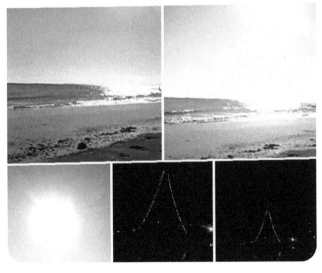

It was a sunset gaze from the Sea Spirit, the last for 2014. What a great day, Happy New Year, everyone.

Sungazing today was at sunset. I experienced frigid temperatures but clear, beautiful blue skies.

January 9, 2015 (thirty-nine minutes)

Leo Walton   •••
Jan 20, 2015 at 4:04 PM • Pinterest • 👥

Hi all...a milestone today...I Sungazed just moments ago...40 min...woowhoo

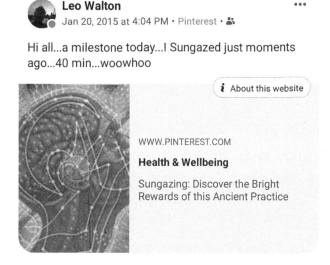

i About this website

WWW.PINTEREST.COM

Health & Wellbeing

Sungazing: Discover the Bright Rewards of this Ancient Practice

I jumped fifteen seconds today instead of ten seconds. I got off by doing the same thing recently.

I made a reference comment about higher consciousness and the positive benefits of sungazing.

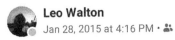

Leo Walton

Jan 28, 2015 at 4:16 PM · 👥

Hi all...Sungazing ...41 minutes...woo...that's a long time...

My goal to complete this phase of the project ends at 44 minutes...

Currently it has taken 11 months to reach this time frame...lots of aggressive Sungazing...not missing an opportunity to gaze...

Another month and I'll be done with phase one...

Pics...cold hiding from wind on bow of the Spirit beneath canopy...

2nd pics of sun light passing through colored jars filled with water and a clear quartz crystal inside...

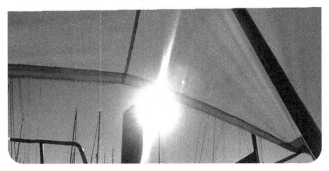

January 20, 2015 (forty minutes)

 Leo Walton
Jan 9, 2015 at 7:33 AM • Pinterest • 👥   •••

As I get closer to reaching my Sungazing goal of 44 mins...my current 39 min capabilities has had many significant positive benefits...

I cannot recommend safe Sungazing enough...

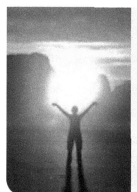

i About this website

WWW.PINTEREST.COM

higher consciousness

Sungazing; isn't it amazing that a simple method of sun-gazing can restore balance and harmony in the mind, body and spirit! There are many proponents of this ancient spiritual technique like the Mayan, ...

Another milestone. I gazed at sunset once more.
Made comment about health and wellbeing.

January 28, 2015 (forty-one minutes)

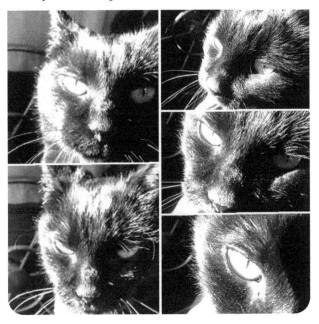

Leo Walton
Jan 11, 2015 at 9:12 AM ·

Always capturing light pics...my cats eyes reveal how the eye absorbs light...

Currently, it has taken eleven months to reach this duration of time sungazing. Another month I'm predicting I will be finished with the HRM Protocol.

February 7, 2015 (forty-three minutes)

Wow, just one more minute to finish this experiment. I referenced info on pineal gland and chemical production.

February 12, 2015 (forty-three minutes forty-five seconds)

I'm sprinting to the finish line. It was a beautiful, calm, frigid day again at sunset.

February 13, 2015 (forty-four minutes)

Awesome project, and it is now officially complete. I have met all the requirements of sungazing time requirements of the HRM Protocol.

I am very pleased to complete this project and also at the same time sorry to see it end. It has been hands-down one of the greatest experiences of my lifetime.

I want to think my guru, Hira Ratan Manek, for his years of research, experimentation, and tenacious engagement in promoting sungazing.

If it were not for his championship efforts, honesty, and compassionate efforts, I do not believe I would be writing this text to attempt to contribute my part to getting this information published. I'll never forget the e-mail he forwarded to me when I contacted him to tell him I was using his methods and lecturing on them in workshops.

HRM said, "Tell the world about sungazing, tell them all!"

Thanks, Hira, I'm trying my best.

Leo Walton
Feb 7, 2015 at 4:13 PM • Pinterest • 👥

Hi all Sungazing 43 min today...just 1 min to go...

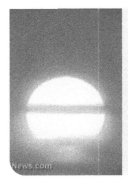

WWW.PINTEREST.COM

Just Stuff

Enhanced production of melatonin and serotonin - Research has found when direct sunlight enters the eyes, it moves through the retinal hypothalamic tract and continues into the brain. The pineal gland is th...

Leo Walton
Feb 21, 2015 at 8:55 PM • 👥

Wendy took this shot the day I hit 44 mins Sungazing...

Look close you can see the sunglasses have holes in the lens...

Look real close you can see my pupils...

Lol...

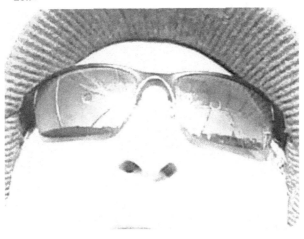

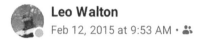

Leo Walton
Feb 12, 2015 at 9:53 AM · 👥

Morning all...Sungazing 43 min 45 sec...

Beautiful and cold but calm...

Sunset from yesterday... Had to post again...

One of the best photos I've taken in a while...

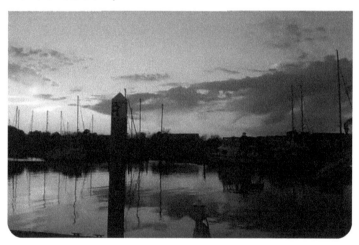

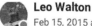

Leo Walton   •••
Feb 15, 2015 at 7:25 AM • Pinterest • 👥

Morning all...Friday 13th was the perfect date to complete my nearly year long research project of Sungazing...

I reached the 44 min goal and will not need to ever sun gaze again...unless I choose...

I don't believe I will ever stop...

Anyway this journey had so many positive benefits I am 90 pages into a new book detailing my experiences...

Over all...it required 90 hours of starring at the sun...it took 260 sunny days spanning over 350 day time frame...

My wife Wendy has managed to reach 20 min of gaze time...which is an incredible feat...

As with the completion of a project...I sometimes am saddened by the accomplishment...

Its always about the journey...never the destination...

I must admit though...

This has been a journey I will never forget...

Chapter 12

Summation Phase 3: Healing of Spirit, Soul, Achieving Homeostasis, Enlightenment, and Solar Nutrition, and Completion of the HRM Protocol

It has taken fifteen days shy of a year, three hundred fifty days total, of aggressive sungazing experiences since March 1, 2014, when I started at ten seconds duration gaze time, to reach forty-four minutes sungazing duration on February 13, 2015.

I spent two hundred sixty days accumulating a total of ninety hours that I physically spent staring at the sun to fulfill the forty-four minutes total ability to stare at the sun.

This means that seventy-five days of the sungazing opportunities were not possible due to weather or other unfavorable conditions, such as the insect invasion I mentioned before.

I also made eighty-eight posts about my sungazing experiences on my Facebook page, including images and updates to how long I gazed and the current weather conditions. Some of the images are spectacular, and I am including many in this publication to allow my readers the opportunity to witness my experiences of this great endeavor. One of the images will be used for the book cover that will be published from this manuscript.

The results so far have eliminated hunger from my life. It is amazing to never feel hungry, and I can go three days fasting without any cravings. Another thing I've experienced is the lack of satiation when I eat; in other words, I don't feel full anymore. The only feelings are physical—belly empty, belly full—none of the typical sensations I'm accustomed to feeling to make me desire food or to stop eating when I do.

I'm finding some days I only eat one meal, and other times I don't feel the urge to eat everything on my plate, so I'm eating less calories overall.

The hair on my head is growing longer and has filled in my bald area.

My sleep patterns are normal. Still no occurrence of night sweats since they ended.

It has now been a year since I have needed a spinal injection for pain from my herniated disc. This is a miracle to me. I had an appointment with my back surgeon and explained to him my improvements and that I believed that my herniated disc had shrunk back into its proper place. His response was laughing out loud.

One day, I will have an MRI and see the physical evidence and so will he. I don't know when that will occur, I'm pain free now, and an MRI is not warranted.

My life has elevated to a higher frequency overall. I feel good, sleep good, and pain free—how can you do better than that?

It all seems so surreal now to even think I considered doing such an experiment with so much negative information I've been told my entire life.

I can speak from experience and claim with authority the data is all lies and misinformation that is intentional to keep us sick and dumb. The elite few that control the earth do not want healthy, enlightened, and a free-thinking public.

I am proud of the accomplishment, but it is the heart of winter, and the influence of the sun is weaker now. Based on this fact alone, I have made a decision to add one more minute of gaze time to the forty-four minutes of the program to make it forty-five minutes.

(Note: I have also determined that the lessening of my cataracts on my eyes was most likely a combination of sunrays and the sun's heat; therefore, I have decided to continue a second experiment as well. This second experiment is beyond the scope of the HRM Protocol, and I will do it cautiously, feeling confident that I can recognize from experience when the sun is safe to gaze. I do not recommend anyone try this experiment.)

Chapter 13

The Cataracts Experiment

With this particular experiment, I will be shorter in describing. My reasons are first, I'm not going for duration increases to achieve a new personal record of my capabilities. All gazes are exactly forty-five minutes duration.

Secondly, I wasn't trying to experiment with any methods to see boundaries of energy fields and streams. I was consistent with highest priority—heat from sun to dissolve cataract proteins, with simple gazing methods and techniques I had learned as well.

Thirdly, all gazes were with the new designed sungazing glasses I had created.

(Note: I thought of manufacturing these glasses for about a minute's time.)

My visit with one optometrist who tested the glasses under many different examination methods and equipment, including a self-test using his own eyes as a measurement system, once he had performed the measurements, he had the capabilities, plus mapping each one on paper, thus documenting the exact specifications used and as designed, answering the questions I came there with.

Then after completing the task I had contracted him for, he had some very technical questions himself.

His inquiry based on pure curiosity was splendid.

He could not believe how much his vision was improved wearing them to read his own charts, compared to what he had been using for decades.

Also, he was wearing his own prescription glasses, which he removed for eye exam.

Basically, he used his own system he uses on patients to run a barrage of testing on my design to check it for accuracy.

His summation was that I should immediately apply for a US patent on these glasses and this design.

That really makes your confidence grow.

However, the precision and skill that is required to manufacture these glasses, they are and should be customized same as any prescription with routine visits to monitor progress.

I designed the glasses to provide not only protection to the eye organ from reflective glare but also to guarantee that pupil gaze holes are as perfect as possible within several thousands of tolerances.

It should all be medically followed and tested. It would be as critical as using an optometrist to make in prescription form.

My vote is, honestly, this is the route sungazing and optometry need to unite together in order to provide great health and healing benefits for mankind.

The optometrist organization has an opportunity and should include desire to do the best things for you to improvement not only eye health but help balance all systems to a healthy, long life. It's sad it is not that way now, but it can be.

The optometrist is the most trained to measure the effects of sungazing is having on your eyes. This is critical. It's very important. I had three different ones and a prescription from my longest and first optometrist on this list, who made the determination of lens replacement surgery years before I began sungazing.

I had the first optometrist I visited, who made the recommendation for lens replacement surgery, write the required and tested physician's recommendation and prescription I needed to see the eye surgeon in my health network. I also had two out-of-network optometrists make the same determination for me to have my lenses of my eyes surgically removed and new lenses installed.

I also recommend involving all medical supporters in this experiment. I certainly did in all three of my experiments.

I began this experiment shortly after I reached the forty-five-minute time mark of gazing duration.

On March 1, 2015, I did my first gaze of this experiment. Coincidentally it was exactly one year to the day I had begun the HRM Protocol, on March 1, 2014.

I completed this experiment on September 30, 2015 on the date I made before I began this project.

I have now gazed consistently for nineteen months' time with a total of three hundred forty-four gazes and accumulating a hundred fifty-three hours staring at the sun.

I noticed a significant reduction in the amount of debris accumulation in my eyes in the mornings as I progressed with the longer gaze times.

I also experienced a significant vision change that aided in my determination to see the eye surgeon.

Over the holiday months, I made arrangements to get the proper eye surgeon to schedule a lens transplant on both my eyes at a time that was convenient for me.

At the time, I thought my experiment was a failure.

This is how my appointment went the day with the eye surgeon. I was examined by this physician who had a lengthy list of credentials, including being the head of the local medical board in his field, of my insurance network.

Once he and his associate had completed their series of testing my eyes and he had collected the data of my eyes' condition, he met with me while interfacing with his computer, reviewing the information of his testing.

Our conversation was brief as he turned away from the computer screen and began writing on a pad. He then tore the small page from the pad and handed it to me.

I looked at the information, and to my surprise, it was a prescription for new glasses.

Bewildered and caught off guard, shocked by this unexpected event, I immediately and in a confused manner said, "You do realize I didn't get a prescription from my local optometrist to visit you in another city miles away to get a prescription for eyewear. I came here to schedule lens replacement surgery?" I continued saying, "I had three different optometrists recommend me for lens replacement. I come to you for this procedure, and you give me a prescription for glasses. I don't understand?"

His reply was even more shocking than me receiving a prescription for new glasses. He stated in a very sarcastic way, "It is amazing at how many optometrists are liars out there. I can't do surgery on your eyes because they don't need it. On a cataract rating scale of one to four, with four being the worst, your left eye is zero. It has no evidence of cataracts, and your right eye I would call it a good solid one. Therefore you are not a candidate for lens replacement."

I was so stunned by this conversation and confused that I left his facility with my new glasses prescription and many thoughts firing in my mind.

It was not until later after I had re-examined this event many times that I realized my sungazing experiment had been a huge success.

It was his attitude and demeanor about the integrity of his colleagues, including the one in his own network of providers that recommended him, that really threw me a curve ball.

In hindsight, he was aware I had been experimenting with sungazing and was dead against the method. I can only believe him so egotistical to deny obvious physical evidence that sungazing actually eliminated the cataracts. He chose to demean his colleagues and their professionalism rather than accept hard facts that went against his belief system—or possibly his self-defense of economic loss? I don't know.

I feel sorry for people that so many lies exist in the medical industry.

Therefore, in conclusion, I have to accept the belief that my experiment was a phenomenal success. The reason my vision changed so dramatically was because the proteins which constitute the composition in my cataracts had dissolved from the sun.

Chapter 14

Ninety Days No Food Experiment, Solar Nutrition

Following my nineteen months of magnificent sungazing experiments, I continued to perform short-duration gazes and walking barefoot on the beach as a routine.

HRM states,

> As you mature with gazing at the Sun, you reach transitional stages. When it comes to hunger, typically at 30 minutes time frame of starring at the Sun, is the average for most gazers to experience, the Sungazer begins to lose the desire to eat. Hunger pains completely diminish, cravings begin to fade away and the desire to eat becomes less and less of a priority.

I couldn't agree more with HRM on this process.

As I stated earlier in this text, I completed all sungazing experiments on September 30, 2015, and as a result, I experienced no more hunger. Even a lack of desire to eat became the norm. I became increasingly less interested in eating anything and began to seriously consider doing more than a three-day fast, which I was doing often.

When I was performing my sungazing experiments, I noticed at around twenty minutes that I started experiencing a decreased desire to eat.

At that time, I was already a practicing vegetarian, which in my opinion, as well as HRM, is the natural transition and should be a lengthy one to train the body to be free of food.

HRM says, "The reason this method is critical, is the transition should be simple, easy, and not stress the body to the extent, that many do achieve, this skill of being able to survive without eating."

(*Note: HRM stopped eating in 1995 and has been examined by several in depth studies. One he was examined in India for four hundred eleven days by an entire team of doctors. Another experiment, he was examined for twenty-four hours a day, for a hundred days in America by a team of researchers at the University of Pennsylvania. Reportedly they were contracted by NASA to use for long-term space voyages, such as sending a man to Mars. The results of the final conclusion presented was that HRM did survive largely on sunlight. They claimed that Hira only consumed an occasional small amount of water or buttermilk the entire time.*)

The water HRM consumes is distilled—that is, solar-imprinted or plasma-infused.

Breatharian is another term used, and an Australian author of *Food of the Gods,* who goes by the name of Jasmuheen, had a twenty-one-day program she promoted to stop eating. This program shocks the body from eater to non-eater. She had a high failure rate for those who did her program who continued being non-eaters for very long, and there were some accidental deaths associated with her program, where people had put themselves in isolated areas to implement her program. The results were they became too weak to be capable of getting themselves to emergency help. I understand she has stopped this method and has another procedure to follow.

More recently, Ray Maor from Israel has developed a shorter ten-day, no-food program, which includes a four-day water fast period at the same time. He wrote a book recently about going for a year as a non-eater. He claims a high success rate using his method, and his graduates continue for months or years after his initiation as non-eaters.

Ray has a recent book about his experiences titled *A Year Without Food.*

I call both these methods the shotgun approach and from experience can claim that the sungazing route to becoming a non-eater is a natural approach that is gradual, gentler, and much kinder program.

(*Note: at the time I began my ninety days as a non-eater, my body was well trained with two years as a sungazer, several years as a vegetarian, and I often did twenty-four-hour and three-day fasts, so I was living this lifestyle for some time and was accustomed. Just a little trick I learned on fasting that makes it easier to perform in the beginning. Try beginning your fast after you eat your evening meal of the day. This way, your sleep is not disturbed by an empty stomach and hunger pains from going all day with no food. For example, you eat at 6:00 p.m., when you awaken in the morning at 6:00 a.m., you have already successfully completed 50 percent (twelve hours) of your twenty-four-hour fast effortlessly.*)

On December 5, 2016, a little more than a year from completing the sungazing experiments, I was eating an egg, mushroom, onion, and cheese quesadilla at 7:00 p.m. in the evening—the only thing I'd eaten that day.

I couldn't eat it. After about half-way, I frustratingly said, "I'm done, I'm going to stop eating today. This is my last meal till whenever."

I already had been researching different breatharian and solar nutritional methods including years of creating and consuming my *"rainbow water,"* calculating the math over the months preceding to develop how many calories the body required for maintaining metabolic functions and how I could create a scale to understand what I could take in and how.

Other than air, for me, it was going to be basically two sources of fuel—short-duration sungazes and my *"rainbow water."*

I haven't mentioned before now, but during my Giza Pyramids research, I had figured out how the systems functioned there and how the pyramids themselves were used to influence the water that was circulated between them and the other systems below the ground.

I had been researching, experimenting, and I began manufacturing this *"rainbow eater,"* I call it, from distilled water that takes two days to complete and consuming it for a couple years prior. I already knew it had a high-energy caloric capacity.

(Note: I have a chapter to follow on how to make this magnificent water yourself as a part of this book.)

Let's take a few minutes to go over my calculations I had determined prior to beginning my ninety-day fast on December 5, 2016.

Years ago during my earlier research, I studied the great works of Austrian naturalist, Viktor Schauberger, known as the "water wizard," and became intrigued by his experiments and conclusions.

Viktor's son, Walter, was also a part of his father's research and became an engineer who used his knowledge of mathematics to calculate energy formulas to complement his dad's theories.

I used some of Walter's formulas in my search for data to understand what I was planning to do with regards to energy calories.

I figured up so many different calculations, attempting to create a simple method to explain the sun's energies in the same way as if eating a food source based on calories.

I'll compare the difference in a vegetarian diet versus a meat diet to present a baseline.

The vegetarian diet provides a well-balanced pH level in their blood system and has mostly alkaline in nature, ranging below seven on the pH scale. Digestion is simple, fast, and produces efficient waste excrement.

However, if you consume red meat, chicken, or pork, extra physical work is necessary by the body to digest, and the blood pH levels are acidic, above seven on the pH scale.

1. The demand for water is increased.
2. The production of hydrochloric acid is increased significantly to aid in digesting the meat, therefore making the blood more acidic.
3. Eating meat require three times the amount of time to digest and longer to excrete as waste, an average of eighteen hours versus six for vegetarian.

Therefore, one recommendation I learned before stopping to eat and beginning a solar nutritional program is changing to a vegetarian diet in preparation.

(Note: some food sources are better energy suppliers than others. As a matter of fact, many processed foods require more energy to digest and excrete than they provide in energy to accomplish. It's why it's called junk.)

I even calculated the cost of the food, how many hours of work had to be performed to pay for it, driving to shop for it, electricity to cook it, and time to prepare, eat and clean up afterwards—it is amazing when you figure how much of our lives center around food.

Before I could calculate, there was some general scientific information available which I gathered to share.

1. The human body's metabolism requires 8 to 10 percent of an individual's energy expenditure.
2. Physical activity is an average depending on activity level is typical of between 20 and 30 percent of energy expenditure.
3. If you work out in addition, that work would need calculating and add the post exercise increase in metabolic demand by 15 percent more.

The MET system is a sliding scale of one to twelve. Light to heavy is offered.

Here is a sample break down I discovered from the Spear Madsen researchers who chemically tested thousands upon thousands of individuals from professional athletes to elderly grandmothers.

It is widely agreed by medical science, two thousand calories, the average calories consumed by a woman, and two thousand five hundred by a man within twenty-four hours to maintain their current mass.

I decided to choose a simple number to use to simplify explanation, so I chose two thousand four hundred calories, breaking it down to a hundred calories an hour for a twenty-four-hour day.

100 calories an hour = 2400 a day
10% for metabolic = 10 calories per hour x 24 = 240 calories
25% for physical = 25 calories per hour x 24 = 600 calories

15% for post exercise = 15 calories per hour x 24 = 360 calories
50% of calories needed/50 calories per hour x 24 = 1200 calories

Therefore, twelve hundred calories a day is the average minimum caloric intake needed to handle all metabolic functions, including typical physical exertion required for a typical daily requirement.

My questions became about how many energy calories can a man get from the sun and how many energy calories my *"rainbow water"* provides.

I got to thinking about the calories I could save by not consuming food at all. No fuel or calories needed for digestion and none for simulation or excretions of waste. I could eliminate all of these power drains by not eating.

So if I'm eating 2400 calories a day and I stop eating and I only need 1200 calories a day, that means 50 percent of the calories I consume a day go just for the mechanics of eating alone.

Wow! That doesn't appear to be a very efficient energy system when 50 percent of everything we eat is used just to accommodate our eating system, and that is when we eat only high-quality foods.

When you look at eating from this perspective, at the onset, it leaves a lot to be desired. However, my research has discovered some interesting variables to be included.

I had been doing routine three-day fast and drinking my "rainbow water," as well as monitoring my energy levels for a lengthy period of time—including performing short duration sungazes lasting no longer than ten minutes. Since I completed both my sungazing projects, I had a generalized idea that I was getting a significant amount of energy as calories using these two techniques.

My investigation into measuring the energy of my solar-infused water and the direct energy I was receiving from the sun, which included the surrounding environment, I put together this method as a general guideline.

With my passionate bio-energetics research being an on-going project, the foundation many of my theories were based upon, I had already spent years testing different electromagnetic energy streams, additional earth telluric currents, the sun's energies including specialized ancient tools influence and effects they had on the human bodies energy systems.

I'm including three drawings that offer a visual representation.

When you consider sun energy, it is currently scientifically calculated on the sun's power per square meter of earth. That's about thirty-nine inches square.

My research concluded that the average human energy field is the source where the ancient cubit of measurement was created to represent. This is about twenty and a half inches cubed, and I titled it the Cubit of Man—which if we take these two shapes, the "Cubit of Man" fits perfectly inside the one square meter of solar energy influence.

What I am about to describe is similar in concept as these new cellphone charging grids that you just lay your phone on top of it, and it charges your cellphone wirelessly.

Of course, when dealing with the sun's energy, I had to come up with a system that I could use and be able to measure differences in the energy amounts. For example, different latitude and the seasons of the year, winter versus summer, all have a solar minimum and solar maximum range.

I purposely used a couple familiar energy categories out of necessity and have made some interesting calculations to make it understandable at the end. I've used watts and calories because of the difference between sunlight measurement and human measurement but have coupled them in a way I hope you can understand.

I've often quoted the average wattage of the human body produces the same energy as the electricity needed to keep a single hundred-watt lightbulb burning for one hour. Multiply with twenty-four, that equals two thousand four hundred watts for each day.

Here is how that is calculated:

A hundred-watt lightbulb burning continuously for twenty-four hours converts to calories this way. The math formula is two multiplied by ten to the sixth power equals calories per day.

Breaking this down for the non-math-minded person, it works like this:

$$2 \times (10 \times 10 \times 10 \times 10 \times 10 \times 10) = 2 \times (1,000,000) = 2,000,000$$

That's two million calories.

Using this conversion now sheds new light on the human body's magnificent abilities of energy expenditure from a different perspective. The average human has the incredible ability of producing a hundred times the effort of the calories that we consume from food, so this is explained in this way.

I will use for calculation two thousand calories of our daily diet calories in this exercise.

Therefore, two thousand multiplied by a hundred—that's two million calories, the same exact energy amount to burn the hundred-watt lightbulb for twenty-four hours.

I wish I could take credit for this data, but scientists beat me to it.

I find this type of data fascinating and plan to use it often when calculating human energy.

Now let us return to the measurements of sun energy per square meter of earth we mentioned previously—the "earth grid charger," I will name it.

To create a baseline, I decided to use sun data collected from forty degrees latitude—what is known as the fortieth parallel. This is a circle of latitude north of the earth's equatorial plane. It crosses Europe, the Mediterranean Sea, Asia, the Atlantic, the Pacific and the North American continent.

At this latitude, the sun is visible for fifteen hours and one minute on summer solstice and nine hours and twenty minutes on winter solstice. In June, the sun is 73.83 degrees and in December is at 26.17 degrees—a huge difference on energy intensity and strength.

Using fifteen hours of sunlight for summer and nine hours of Sunlight for winter, we can create an accurate measurement between the two seasons to create a solar maximum (summer) and solar minimum (winter) baseline.

By doing so, we will have a better understanding of energy human energy management.

I broke the information down to one-hour increments for simplification.

In the summer, the sun at forty degrees provides six hundred watts of energy to one square meter of earth per hour. That means the energy produced would be equal to six multiplied with hundred-watt bulbs for that small sample of earth every hour, and there are fifteen hours of sunlight—astounding.

In the winter, the sun at forty degrees. Same location provides three hundreds watts of energy. This is a 50 percent reduction in energy production and explains why the leaves fall from the trees and vegetable gardens cannot flourish. Therefore in winter, the same square meter of earth only equals to three multiplied with hundred-watt bulbs.

I went further in this relationship by associating my forty-five-minute sungazing experiments while standing in the one square meter of earth grid and using my "cubit of man" analogy, which is exactly what you are doing when you sungaze.

That meant every minute of time was equal to being bombarded by ten watts of energy from the sun; therefore, in forty-five minutes, it would have been four hundred fifty watts of energy available to utilize in the summertime or only two hundred twenty-five watts during the winter.

From scientific conversion charts focusing on a calorie aspect:

450 watts = 1620 kilo calories
225 watts = 810 kilo calories

That is a lot of energy that the human body is capable of tapping into—once he has trained his systems to integrate with it by attunement from sungazing.

It is quite remarkable the superhuman capabilities of the human body that we have lost over time.

It's obvious that sungazing allows us to tap into this huge quantity of energy, but I want to comment further on the energy from my "rainbow water."

Over the years, I guesstimated I was receiving about 30 percent of my caloric energy requirements from my water alone.

So when I started looking at the results of all this data collection, I knew by not eating, my body would not need twelve hundred calories of my typical twenty-four hundred-calorie requirements. This meant with twelve hundred calories, my new target, my water at 30 percent reduced the need of three hundred sixty calories (1200 − 360 = 840 calories).

So my ten-minute sungazes had to equal eight hundred forty calories to make me meet the necessary caloric requirements to survive without food.

Sounds impossible, doesn't it?

But there is a little more to the story. As a mature sungazer and according to HRM's research and recommendations, once you reach forty-four minutes, you never need to sungaze ever again. Your body has become so attuned that only an occasional few minutes of being in the sun will charge your systems.

In my experiments over the years, my determination is this: once you have attuned your bio-energy systems to the sun, the detoxification of your pineal gland allows you the ability to super charge its function capabilities. This attunement and calibration does more than restrict your energy requirements to a few methods. Once you are a mature, trained sungazer, your energy systems become flexible and develops the abilities to maximize all energy systems cosmically and earthly.

You become a perfect example of energy management, utilizing quantum entanglement of all energies, and gain the ability to provide caloric energy intake, fueling the human body from all energy sources—true freedom.

This transformation is incredible and simple to obtain and is the true representation of "illumination."

With the abundance of our energy sources available to all life on the planet, the sun, man doesn't need much solid food.

Now that we have a better understanding of how all this works, I want to describe the experiences of going ninety days with no food.

CHAPTER 15

THE INCREDIBLE JOURNEY

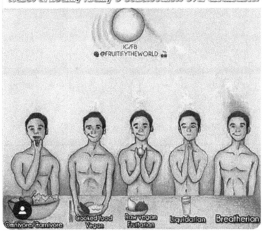

The lighter foods thy eat, the lighter thy shall be. One step at a time, through un-fooding you can reach the highest states of health, vitality & conciousness ever attainable.

IG/FB
@ @FRUITIFYTHEWORLD

Omnivore/Carnivore | Cooked food Vegan | Raw vegan Fruitarian | Liquidarian | Breatherian

Before I undertake the significant details related to my ninety days of non-eating, I want to speak a little more about our breath as an energy-gathering mechanism and add some more critical data about the sun from other resources.

Different cultures all have their names they call the breath. The Hebrews call it *ruah*, "breath of life," the Hindus and Buddhist call it "prana," and the Chinese call it "chi."

Practices such as yoga, sun-do, gigu, and pranic breathing all incorporate abdominal breathing techniques to cleanse and invigorate the body.

More prana is absorbed with slow deep breaths than shallow breathing. The average human breath should be six times per minute, but most humans breathe twelve to twenty times per minute. At these rates, we are not collecting the ambient energy that's available and our bodies require to function at its best.

As we showed in the equations earlier, the amount of prana being emitted from the sun is beyond our comprehension.

On December 5, 2016, I made the decision to stop eating food. I didn't know at that moment when I would take my next bite of solid food again. At the onset, I thought I would attempt to go one year's duration, but that wasn't a firm commitment.

I already knew that the sun's position in the sky was getting further away from my physical location as we got closer to winter solstice. This one issue was my greatest concern that the sun would not be strong enough to adequately provide the essential vitamins, minerals, and essential amino acids that form the proteins necessary for survival from gazing at the sun.

At this time, my research wasn't as complete on understanding the energy formulas I detailed earlier, but I had learned from my cataract experiment the significance the sun's intensity differences between summer and winter seasons.

Most people do not understand the food chain and how our diet is created by the sun.

It is easy to see if you live in some latitudes that experience the four seasons of the year—spring, summer, fall, and winter—and recognize the effect the sun's distance from earth influences the plant life, from the leaves on the trees to the periods when vegetables will grow and the flowers bloom.

It affects many species of birds and fish who migrate south to warmer waters and temperatures.

A brief explanation is the sun's energy changes when it comes into contact with our atmosphere. An alchemy between the frequencies create all the vitamins, minerals, amino acids, and proteins needed to support the life forms on earth.

These nutritional building blocks are basically planted into the topsoil of the earth, which acts like a sponge that absorbs the nutrients.

A plant will grow and thrive by using water as a medium to suck these nutrients into its root systems, then the sun creates a capillary action causing the nutrients to spread throughout the entire plant and any fruit it may produce.

These plants contain the full spectrum of nutrition humans and most animals need to survive and thrive on earth. Man became a carnivore over time by eating the animals that get their nutrition from eating the plants, which is a weaker and diluted source of nutrition, but during seasons that do not produce vegetation, man learned he could survive these periods by eating the animals.

Therefore, man only required meat to survive harsh cold environments, learning to have a flexible diet based on the food sources availability.

The animals receive much better quality of minerals, vitamins, and proteins from the plants than man does eating the remnants of the plants after the animals process it into their flesh, then we cook it, reducing the quality even further.

So when you think back to my earlier statements about the eighteen hours it requires of energy and acid environment inside your body, eating meat, some worse than others, isn't logical or beneficial, unless there is no other food source, and it becomes a matter of survival.

So back to December 5, I made the decision to drink coffee, tea, and my "rainbow water" as my only intake other than sungazing.

I also began to calculate when I should schedule a physical with my primary physician to measure my progress.

For the first several days, I never noticed any significant changes until days four or five. I began to miss the act of chewing. It was really an odd occurrence. I've always liked crunchy things like nuts, apples, celery, popcorn, potato chips, and the like—even hard candies.

I did recognize my trips to the toilet were becoming less frequent, and I had less waste to excrete.

By the second week without food, I was craving chewing, not food but the act of chewing. I purchased some chewing gum and tried for a few days to calm the urge, but it did not meet the satisfaction for something crunchy.

I quickly learned how a rat must feel that needs to gnaw constantly on all types of hard things to retard the growing of their front teeth. The desire to chew was incessant.

I then decided to take one almond nut and chew it with my front teeth, taking minutes to do so and then spitting out the contents rather than swallowing. I performed this routine many times a day for another week, and oddly enough, the sensations to chew left, so I halted this method, and the desire to chew never returned.

It is amazing at how the body and mind is so determined to get you to consume solid food.

By the third week, my bowl movements were between three and four days a part. It was around this time I was curious why I had bowl movements at all because I wasn't consuming anything to excrete, and it finally became clear. The raw cocoa I was putting into my three or four cups of coffee a day for flavor was an indigestible fiber, and it became visually obvious this was the only product I was excreting.

Once my body had adjusted to the lack of chewing demands, I became more relaxed and focused.

I began to enjoy the lack of food. I noticed my sleep requirements reduce significantly. Ultimately I was sleeping between two hours and four hours a night and would awaken wide awake and energetic, so I researched the chemical process that occurs to the body when a human stops consuming food.

What I discovered was short of fantastic, while we understand that the pineal gland produces the hormone melatonin. By not eating, the endocrine system operates at its maximum capacity. Also, literally without food products and waste products circulating through our bodies and the demands placed upon it, the 50 percent of calories we eat to fulfill these processes, the increase efficiency of melatonin production is a higher quality because it is not diluted by other chemicals and products from eating.

The result was a peaceful attitude and a relaxed emotional frequency that made the entire day joyful. It was like being in a conscious meditative state all the time.

Another chemical that is produced in greater abundance and has a significant effect on your state of being is the increase in DMT levels. DMT stands for dimethyltryptamine and is the human's production of a hallucinogenic chemical compound similar to LSD that naturally forms in some plants and mushrooms. The DMT elevates you to a very euphoric frame of mind your entire waking cycle.

As I stated earlier, I was only sleeping two to four hours a night, and I worked frantically the entire time. I never was tired, felt great, and had more energy to the point where I was the most mentally alert and physically strong and active as any time in my life.

It was an incredible existence.

During the entire ninety days of non-eating, I continued my exercise routine—my three- to four-mile walks most days, riding my bicycle sometimes multiple times a day, yoga, and a few strength exercises.

Speaking of strength, I did notice a loss of strength when doing some things that required physical exertion, such as lifting heavy things and such, but I attributed most of it to the fact that I ended up losing forty pounds of body weight. I went from a hundred seventy pounds to a hundred thirty pounds, reducing my waist size from thirty-six inches to thirty inches—the same size as when I graduated high school in 1971.

I noticed an atrophy in muscle size, and the physical appearance of my face lost all subcutaneous fat, which made my face withdrawn, my eyes were sunken, and to me, unhealthy-looking, but I felt amazing.

As a matter of fact, I took a selfie of myself 100 percent by accident near the end of my ninety days, and it was months afterwards I had done so. I saw a post on Facebook someone posted the last image of Nikola Tesla taken before his death in 1943.

He and I look very similar in facial characteristics and expression, it was unsettling and uncanny. I have included the two images for you to witness for yourself in the chapter upcoming on my discoveries of Tesla being a non-eater and sungazer.

Believe me, neither images are very flattering.

Seventy-five days into my non-eating experiment, I met with my primary physician, who performed a complete physical including blood work which included testing of proteins.

It took two weeks for me to get the results of all the testing. During the exam and my conversation with the doctor, who has been a great supporter of my experiments over the years and also the person I eventually ended up with as a result of my NDE from my electrocution, she asked me how I would react to the test results if unfavorable. I made a promise to her then that I would return to eating to resolve the problems. She was on board 100 percent after that verbal contract.

I am a miracle man to her already, she told me a while back. She stated that in her thirty years of experience, the only people she had examined following an electrocution similar to mine, she had to remove the white sheet from atop their corpse to view. She has also been a part of my sungazing experiments and has never known anyone who has stared at the sun naked-eyed like I have. Now I was there after going seventy-five days with no food.

When I received the results of the testing, it was day eighty-nine of my non-eating experiment.

The results showed my heart perfect, my blood pressure was perfect, my respiration perfect, my cholesterol perfect, my vitamins perfect, and my minerals perfect.

(Note: I want to remind everyone that prior to my sungazing experiments I was on six different prescription drugs for a plethora of issues, seven for a short duration due to swelling a symptom caused by one of the medications prescribed. Now my physical data is perfect and drug-free.)

I was 10 percent deficient in protein levels, the only problem with having aced the entire exam.

Before I began the non-eating fast, I already knew that HRM consumed small amounts of buttermilk, the only food source he has in taken for years.

My blood test revealed to me that protein is the hardest to ingest from the sun particularly in my case because it was winter, and the sun was at its weakest time as I revealed in my calculations—up to 50 percent less energetic at forty degrees latitude. I live at thirty-seven degrees.

I also have known Tesla only consumed buttermilk in his last years. It has been a historical fact reported and documented by a number of researchers and eyewitness accounts.

(*Note: I have always been a big supplement user—vitamins and minerals, super foods, and herbs. I wanted my non-eating test to not be altered by consuming these supplements while doing the experiment, so the results would be pure. This is also why I didn't want to consume buttermilk. Now I know the reasons the ancients and those who have learned directly from like Tesla and my guru HRM make this the single food source they ingest.*)

Today is November 4, 2019 and it has been several years since completing these sungazing and non-eating experiments.

My current status is once I started eating again on March 5, 2017, I went straight to adapting to an intermittent fast. I only consume one meal a day and often a small snack, but I do it in a restricted window of time. I go sixteen to eighteen hours a day with no eating, and I consume my meal and anything I ingest food wise in a six- to eight-hour window of time.

Also, for nearly two years, I modified my diet further, eating a target of twenty-five grams of sugar a day, low carbs, moderate protein, and high-fat diet known as the keto diet.

Between the intermittent fasting and keto diets, I love the systems. They work very well together. I have rocket fuel for energy now that I trained my metabolism to be flexible and able to burn fat rather than just store it. When I say rocket fuel, it is because carbs and proteins are four grams of energy and fat is nine grams. Once you become metabolically flexible, you use fat for fuel, including your own body fat storages, not sugars and carbs.

My weight today has returned to a hundred seventy pounds, and my waist measurements are four inches smaller than when I began my ninety-day experiment at the same weight.

My body fat ratios are significant lower, and I look leaner and more muscular—very good for a sixty-six-year-old man.

I walk about a hundred miles a month and ride my bicycle an average of a hundred fifty miles per month. I am in excellent fitness and health. I cannot recall the last time I have had the flu or a cold.

I can only say my experiments have made huge improvements in every part of my life.

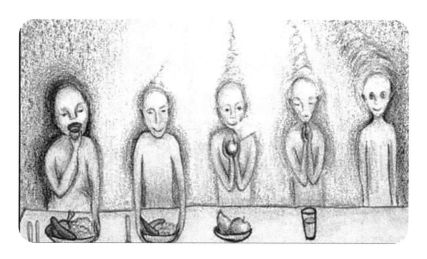

Chapter 16

Nikola Tesla As a Sungazer and Non-Eater

Nikola Tesla (1857 to 1943)

I commented in the introduction to this text on Tesla's interview with journalist John Smith from an interview in 1899. This is a continuation of that topic and begins from an excerpt from Tesla's autobiography he wrote about his own life named "Nikola Tesla's Autobiography, My Inventions." Tesla wrote that while he lived and worked in Budapest, he and his friend, Sigetijem, were walking together in the city park.

As the sun was setting, his friend became concerned because Tesla refused to stop staring at the sun. Following several failed attempts to verbally distract Tesla's unrelenting gaze, his friend physically grabbed Tesla, trying to force him to look away from the sun. Tesla, refusing to turn his head away from the sun, struggled with his friend who was trying desperately to get him to look away. Suddenly, Tesla reached down and, grabbing a stick off the ground, began drawing the working blueprints for AC electricity generators in the dirt, all the while exclaiming excitedly, "I can see it! I can see it! I can see it how it works! I can see how it rotates in different directions and oscillates."

Continuing with the interview with Mr. Smith, Tesla stated confidently, "I am part of a light, and it is the music. The light fills my six senses; I see it, hear, feel, smell, touch and think. Thinking of it…means my sixth sense."

(Note: If you aren't familiar with Tesla and don't have an understanding, of the meanings behind these words, I'll explain.)

During the interview with John Smith, Tesla simply said that he was psychic, as if the interview were a casual conversation with a close friend. Tesla went on to say, "Particles of light are a written note. A bolt of lightning can be an entire sonata. A thousand bolts of lightning, is a concert."

When Smith questioned Tesla concerning world problems, Tesla replied, "One issue, was food, what a Stellar or Terrestrial energy, to feed the hungry on Earth?" *(Stellar means star. Both our sun and Sirius are stars. When he speaks of terrestrial energy, it's not just earth energy he is referencing, it's our four terrestrial planets including our own satellite, the moon, Mars, Venus, and Mercury.)*

(Note: Now we have two different sources with Tesla telling the same story. My determinations on what I understand by becoming a trained sungazer and having hundreds of hours of maturity to source from. I can say without a doubt that Nikola Tesla had to be at least an intermediate sungazer to be able to stare directly at the sun. It requires the ability to stare naked-eyed at the sun for many minutes duration to attune the rods and cones of the eyes to tolerate the intensity of the sun's energies. Also, the entire optic pathways including the hypothalamus, which is like a mirror that reflects the sun's light upon the pineal gland, requires attunement to these same frequencies as well. Only after adequate training of these visual centers would Tesla have been able to witness the intense and dynamic energy fields rotating, pulsing, and oscillations, including phase shifts of these frequencies in order to pick up a stick and draw the first detailed blueprints of the very first alternating current generator motor in the dirt in Istanbul.)

From here, I'd like to discuss Nikola Tesla's relationship with the Eastern Hindu Vedic system and his close friendship with one of the first western world influences from this sect, Swami Vivekananda.

Swami Vivekananda was born in 1863 in Kolkata, India just six years after Tesla. He died a young man in 1902 at the age of thirty-nine. In that time, he had become an Indian Hindu monk and a chief disciple of the nineteenth century Indian Mystic Ramakrishna. He became extremely popular in the Western world and an instant success in the United Kingdom and United States of American when he published his book titled *Raja Yoga* in 1896 which was his interpretation of Patanjali's immortal classic of the yoga Sutra's.

(Note: as a trained yogi who has adapted to a Vedic lifestyle, I have read both of these great text as I believe Nikola Tesla did as well.)

According to an article written by Subash Kak, on February 13, 1896, Vivekananda wrote a letter in response to meeting Tesla at the party actress Sarah Bernhardt had thrown, which both gentlemen attended and engaged in scientific discussion.

The Swami stated that "Mr. Tesla was charmed to hear about the Vedantic Prana and Akasha and the Kalpas. He thinks he can demonstrate mathematically that force and matter are reducible to potential energy. I am to go see him next week to get this mathematical demonstration. In that case Vedantic cosmology will be placed on the surest of foundations. I clearly see their perfect union with modern science, and the elucidation of one will be followed by that of the other."

(Note: a brief description of these three Vedic Hindu Sanskrit words: Prana is the breath or "life force" which permeates reality on all levels including inanimate objects such as stones. It is described as originating from the sun and connects to the elements. There are five categories of Prana described in the texts with Pranayama being one of the eight limbs of yoga. Akasha is a term used to describe either open space or aether in traditional Indian cosmology. It is considered the basis or essence of all things in the material world, the first element. One translation calls it the "upper sky." Kalpas is a word in Hindu that describes a period of an immense time period. It is assumed as 4,320 million human years and considered to be the length of a single cycle of the cosmos equal to one day of Brahma [God], from creation to dissolution.)

The results of this first meeting between the two, sadly, resulted in a failure by Tesla to be able to demonstrate the equivalence of mass, energy, and time.

It was an Italian named Olinto de Pretto who introduced the formula e=mc2 and made famous by Einstein not long after Vivekananda's pre-mature death.

In 1907, Tesla wrote an article which reflected the influence of Vivekananda called, "Man's Greatest Achievement." He wrote about the use of the Akasha and Prana thus stating,

> [L]ong ago…[mankind] recognized that all perceptual matter comes from a primary substance, or tenuity beyond conception, filling all space, the Akasha or luminiferous aether, which is acted upon by the life giving Prana or creative force, calling into existence, in never ending cycles all things and phenomena. The primary substance, thrown into infinitesimal whirls of prodigious velocity, becomes gross matter; the force subsiding, the motion ceases and matter disappears, reverting to the primary substance.

Both Vivekananda and Tesla were hoping for mutual confirmation of Vedanta physics. That was over a hundred twenty years ago, and the science of physics took an additional thirty more years to develop the framework of quantum physics.

Therefore, it is very obvious, five years following Vivekananda's death, Tesla was very much on the hunt for the answers. He wanted so desperately to prove to his far eastern sage friend who had provided him with so much ancient wisdom.

Let's entertain some other conversations. I'd like to concentrate now on Tesla's experiments with non-eating and his conversion to that lifestyle.

According to author John J O'Neil, who knew Tesla personally and wrote one of the first biographies about Tesla, from excerpts taken from *Prodigal Genius*, published one year after Tesla's death, he made a number of comments about Tesla's diet.

He stated,

> [W]ith the passing decades Tesla shifted away from a meat diet. He substituted fish, always boiled, and finally eliminating the meat entirely, living on a Vegetarian diet. Milk was his main standby and toward the end of his life it was the principal item of diet and it was served warm.

(Note: okay, this is a lifestyle that is exactly what HRM recommended—a Jain Indian and sungazer. It is also the very same path I adapted too as well because it is the natural transition as you become attuned to the frequencies yourself, to the life force energy of our sun. I'm convinced, are you? Tesla, HRM, and I, if we don't include the thousands who have done the same thing over time.)

Tesla published another article in *Century Illustrated Magazine* in June 1900. It was titled, "The Problems of Increasing Human Energy with Special References to the Harnessing of the Sun's Energy."

> A thousand other evils might be mentioned, but all put together, in their bearing upon the problem under discussion, they could not equal a single one, the want of food, brought on by poverty, destitution, and famine. Millions of our enlightened communities, and not with-standing, the many charitable efforts, food, but want of healthful nutriment. How to provide good and plentiful food is, therefore, a most important question of the day. On the general principles the raising of cattle as a means of providing food is objectionable, because, in the since interpreted above, it must undoubtedly tend to the addition of mass of a "smaller velocity." It is certainly preferable to raise vegetables, and I think, therefore vegetarianism is a commendable departure from

the established barbarous habit. That we can subsist on plant food and perform our work even to advantage is not a theory, but well-demonstrated fact. Many races living almost exclusively on vegetables are of superior physique and strength. There is no doubt that some plant food, such as Oatmeal, is more economical than meat, and superior to it in regard to both mechanical and mental performance. Such food, moreover, taxes our digestive organs decidedly less, and, in making us more contented and sociable, produces an amount of good difficult to estimate. In view of these facts every effort should be made to stop the wanton and cruel slaughter of animals, which must be destructive to our morals. To free ourselves from animal instincts and appetites, which keep us down, we should begin at the very root from which we spring: we should effect a radical reform in the character of the food. There seems to be no philosophical necessity for food. We can conceive of organized beings living without nourishment and deriving all the energy they need for the performance of their life-functions from the ambient medium.

(Note: Tesla touched on a lot of points I have already detailed from my own experiences, and the only way to know these things is by experience.)

(Note: again, if you know of Tesla's relationship with Vivekananda, you understand the motives concerning hunger and starvation in India during this period of time. That was the main purpose that prompted Vivekananda to pursue monetary gain from his lectures and writings. He had grown up with poverty and had experienced lengthy fast and countless days without food himself during his lifetime. He was very active and focused on eliminating hunger in his homeland for his people. With this

being said, you can see the common connection between Tesla's comments in this text and Vivekananda's passions for his people's plight.)

In February 1937, Tesla was interviewed by *Liberty Magazine* as told to George Sylvester Viereck, titled "A Machine to End War," where Tesla comments again about eating.

Tesla stated,

> [M]ore people die or grow sick from polluted water than from coffee, tea. Tobacco, and other stimulants. I myself eschew all stimulants. I also practically abstain from meat. The abolition of stimulants will not come by forcibly. It will be no longer fashionable to poison the system with harmful ingredients. Bernarr Macfaden has shown how it is possible to provide palatable food based upon natural products such as milk, honey, and wheat. I believe that the food which is served today in his penny restaurants will be the basis of the epicurean meals in the smartest banquet halls of the twenty-first century. There will be enough wheat and wheat products to feed the entire world, including the teeming millions of China and India, now chronically on the verge of starvation. The earth is bountiful, and where her bounty fails, nitrogen drawn from the air will fertilize her womb. I developed a process for this purpose in 1900.

(Note: there are two comments I want to make about Tesla's statements. First is to explain who Bernarr Macffaden was. He was an American proponent of physical culture, a combination of bodybuilding with the nutritional and health theories. He founded the long running magazine publishing company Macfadden, he is remembered as the "father of the physical culture," and he actually campaigned for the Republican party nomination to run for president. Secondly is Tesla's comments on how nitrogen drawn from the air will fertilize the womb.

More recently, the Keshe Foundation Spaceship Institute, a research facility located in Italy, has been conducting research on lung function and the lung's many systems function for years. He has also studied the method of non-eating called breatharian and explains the processes dealing with how plasma and nitrogen assimilation operates.)

Some additional comments made by Tesla from the same interview with John Smith in 1899 about energy and empty space.

(Note: now that I have introduced a new perspective on Tesla's influences and identified his motivations on some of his own passions, the next series of his comments can be understood from an accurate perspective that many readers and researchers have never understood or have found to be odd enough that many feel Tesla's comments were fabricated.)

Tesla claimed that in the air there existed empty space that was a manifestation of matter that was not awakened. He claimed there was no empty space on this planet nor the universe. He said in black holes, what astronomers speak about, are the most powerful sources of energy and life.

He claimed that first was energy and then came matter. He continues saying,

> What about the birth of the universe? Matter is created from the original eternal energy that we know as light. It shined and the planets, man, and everything on earth and the universe appeared. Matter is an expression of infinite forms of light, because energy is older than it.

Tesla also said that "the human mind cannot comprehend infinity and eternity."

Tesla said, "Man's body is the perfect machine. I know my circuit and what is good for him. The food, that nearly all people eat, to me it is harmful and dangerous."

Continuing, Tesla stated,

> Another method to keep the physical body in shape, the knowledge of how the mental and

vital energies transform into what we want, and we achieve control over all feelings. The Hindus call it Kundalini Yoga. This knowledge can be learned, for what they need many years, or it is acquired at birth. The most of them I acquired at birth. They are in the closest connection with a sexual energy that is the most widespread in the universe. The woman is the biggest thief of that energy, and thus the spiritual power. I've always knew that and was alerted. Of myself I created what I wanted; a thoughtful and spiritual machine.

Tesla stated,

Knowledge comes from space and air, vision is its most perfect set. We have two eyes; earthly and spiritual. It is recommended that they become one eye. The universe then becomes alive and all its manifestations, like a thinking animal. A stone is a thinking sentient being, such as a plant, beast and a man.

(Note: Tesla's comments about spiritual matters including his mention of kundalini energy is a direct reflection of his interpretations of Vivekananda's book, Raja Yoga. *The Sanskrit term* kundalini *in Hinduism is a form of divine energy, sometimes known as the goddess Shakti, believed to be located at the base of the spine, the Muladhara Chakra. It is an important concept in the Vedic Tantra, where it is believed to be a force or power associated with the divine feminine. This energy, when cultivated and awakened through Tantric practice, is believed to lead to spiritual liberation. Kundalini, along with the practices associated with it including kundalini yoga, have been adopted into the Hatha Yoga system since the eleventh century. It has since then been adopted into other forms of Hinduism as well as modern spirituality and New Age thought. The kundalini awakenings have been described as*

occurring by means of a variety of methods, including at birth, as Tesla believed of himself. The kundalini experience is frequently reported to be a distinct feeling of electric current running along the spine. Today, modern Christianity has identified the event and renamed it as the Holy Spirit while degrading and instilling fear toward kundalini.)

(Note: Kundalini awakenings are extraordinary events. If we use the mathematical formulas I introduced earlier, the human energy system is rated at the same as a hundred-watt bulb. An awakened kundalini increases this natural bio-chemical current ten times that amount, equating to a thousand watts. This is the entire design and purpose of yoga. To prepare the nervous system, the lymphatic system and the endocrine system as well as others, to be able to handle the extreme, increase in electric current coursing through out the body. I myself experienced a sudden kundalini awakening in 2007 as a result of my electrocution and NDE from 220-volt, 50-amp AC electricity, which I call my "grand illumination." I now lecture on the topic and am often contacted by those experiencing this phenomena to offer suggestions on dealing with some of the symptoms related to the event. A person who has not prepared their bodies for the event often experience a series of emotional and psychotic complications. It is estimated from some medical studies I've sourced that 30 percent of residents in institutionalized mental facilities in the United States of America are there because of negative symptoms brought on by a sudden kundalini awakening.)

(Note: to elaborate on Tesla's comment about the woman being the biggest thief of this energy, this can be simply explained. Tesla as well as many sages such as Gandhi himself pledge a life of "celibacy." Their beliefs are based on wanting to contain and use this increased energy for spiritual and creative tasks. As with Tesla, he had over three hundred patents and was one of the greatest inventors in history of mankind. He claimed it was his celibacy and respect for his kundalini energy that made him the genius we all benefit from today. In order to contain and internalize this massive current, no sexual relationships can occur, therefore no body fluid loss which contains this vital and divine electricity.)

The journalist Mr. Smith then asked, "What is electricity for you, dear Mr. Tesla?"

Tesla replied,

Everything is electricity. First was the light, endless source from which points out material and distributed in all forms that represent the universe and the earth with all its aspects of life. Black is the true face of light, only we do not see this. It is remarkable grace to man and all creatures. One of its particles that possesses the light, either thermal, nuclear, radiation, chemical, mechanical and an unidentified energy. It has the power to run the earth with its orbit.

Tesla said,

Electricity I am. Or if you wish, I am the electricity in human form. You're electricity too Mr. Smith, but you do not realize it. Man's body and brain are made from a large amount of energy; in me there is a majority of electricity. The energy that is different and everyone is what makes the human eye or soul. For other creatures to their essence, the soul of the plant is a soul of minerals and animals. Brain function and death is manifested in light.

Tesla said,

Everything is light. In one of its rays is the fate of all nations, each nation has its own ray and what great light source do we see in the Sun. And remember, no one who was here did not die. They transformed to the light, and as such exist still. The secret lies in the fact that the light particles restore to their original state.

Mr. Smith asked, "Is this the resurrection?"

Tesla says,

> I prefer to call it a return to a previous energy. Christ and several others knew the secret. I am searching how to preserve human energy. It is forms of light, sometimes straight like heavenly light. I have not looked for it for my own sake, rather for the good of all. I believe my discoveries make people's lives easier and more bearable, and channel them to spirituality and morality.

He continued,

> The first feature of this energy is that it transforms. It is a perpetual transformation, just like clouds. But it is possible to leverage the fact that a man preserves consciousness after the earthly life. In every corner of the universe exist energy of life; one of them is immortality, whose origin is outside of man waiting for him. The universe is spiritual; we are only half that way. The universe is more moral than us, because we do not know his nature and how to harmonize our lives with it.

One of Tesla's greatest interviews—wow!

(Note: To collaborate some of Tesla's statements particularly when he mentioned a process of extracting nitrogen from the air to nourish the earth he designed in 1900, I'm sharing some research data from Dr. Mehran T. Keshe's comments about his ongoing research of sungazing and living without eating food. He is an expert in the field of biology and has a number of theories based on magnetic and gravity influences on the human. He has also provided some of the best theories on human lung function available today where he discusses how nitrogen, oxygen, and plasma are assimilated in the lungs. His work on this topic really supports

Tesla's research on nitrogen as well. Tesla's plan was to use the abundant gas and convert it to another power source. Keshe explains how the lungs do it.)

Nearly all of the earth's atmosphere that we breathe is made up of only five gases: nitrogen is the most abundant at 78 percent, oxygen at 20 percent, water vapor, argon at less than 1 percent, and carbon dioxide at a very low 0.031 percent. Several other compounds are also present in extremely small amounts. Water vapor is listed as the third most abundant gas, and the air can contain as much as 5 percent water vapor but typically ranges between 1 percent and 3 percent.

In the Earth's upper atmosphere, the sun's energy reacting with the gravitational and magnetic fields converts the nitrogen in this plasma space into matter, then the rains collect the nitrogen and bring it to the earth's surface where it becomes food for plant life. This same condition also leads to the production of amino acids as well. When these gases come into contact with the water it produced, this water being in touch with salt, which is the matter out of the earth, they join together to form proteins. The varying salts in the environment convert to forming life on the planet; therefore, life is created from its own condition.

The interesting process that allows humans to survive works the same way regardless if you eat meat or vegetables or energy from the sun. The chemical process which occurs in the stomach from the hydrochloric acid reverts the same matters back to the same elements that entered into the atmosphere from the Sun.

This means the earth system operates same as the lungs; it is all about conversion of the same elements and reverting them back to their original state.

Dr. Keshe says science has been long believed that the red color of our blood is due to the oxygen content, however, Keshe says this is not the case, He says,

> Air comes into our lungs for conversion,
> that the color of our blood is not due to oxygen
> rather its caused by nitrogen, the abundant nitro-

gen releases helium due to the environment pressure and vacuum. If you add the helium to the nitrogen, the two together, then helium becomes a carbon after the nitrogen has been inside you, which is an ionization process that occurs when it interacts with the hydrogen in the lungs. This is why when you breathe out, you release carbon dioxide.

He also comments on how the lungs manufacture water. He states,

> Some of the hydrogen left behind in the lungs after the inhalation is the next stage in the process and it links up with the oxygen, it creates water at the same time and this water lubricates the lungs. It was once believed that water in the lungs was a result of water entering the lungs and that is not the case at all. So, the lungs are moist by the chemical and electrical process that causes a transformation that takes place during this process. Therefore, makes the entire process of water manufacturing inside the lungs totally generated by the breathing process itself.

He continues,

> Science and research has shown repeatedly when you are sick and you get weak, the breathing process changes, the breathing process slows down also sometimes when this happens your lungs sometimes gets filled flooded with liquid. It is not uncommon for a physician to be able to draw between 2 to 3 liters from both lungs and is an extreme amount. When you are sick and those who don't eat, their breathing process slows

down, therefore slow breathing in the body can
absorb this water from the lungs and is the reason
that a person that lives without water.

*(Note: Prahlad Jai is an Indian breatharian monk born in 1929
and has not eaten food or drank water since 1940. He has been studied
in two extensive studies in 2003 and 2010, both headed by Dr. Sudhir
Shah, a neurologist at the Sterling Hospitals in Ahmedabad, India.
He was also involved in the studies performed on Hira Ratan Manek
(HRM), my guru who is the main reason for me to write this text.)*

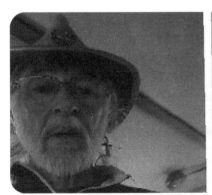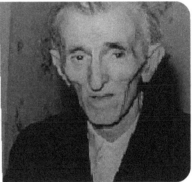

Chapter 17

The Giza Pyramids and My Recipe for Rainbow Water

During my intensive and extensive research on the Giza Plateau and all of the systems there built upon the earth's surface and below the ground (as above/so below), which include the three large pyramids, the Great Pyramid, Kafre, and Menkaure and the six smaller pyramids. Also, there is one pyramid missing known as the Black Pyramid. Ten pyramids in total on the Giza Plateau. Most only believe there were three.

Also, above the ground includes structures such as the Sphinx, the Wall of the Crow, and a number of temples totaling eight. One temple structure, misnamed as a modern structure and not included as being constructed at the same time periods as the others, that sets diagonally in front of the Sphinx makes the total of nine structures.

Below the ground level includes several systems, including Osiris's Tomb, the Cadman Pump a hundred feet below the Great Pyramid, the Tomb of Birds, and three levels of tunnels that act like veins connecting all these systems together into one industrial complex I call Giza Park.

Over a decade of research has allowed my forensics investigator skills, as well as industrial and biological experiences, to complete the most thorough systems analysis of the Giza Plateau since they were constructed.

Please look for my upcoming series of books on describing my theories beginning with *The Giza Park Protocol: How to Start the Sun.*

It was during this research about eight years ago that I discovered how the water that flowed through all the systems were influenced by each structure and how the water reacted to it.

I immediately realized that the water created by this system was powerful, and it helped me realize just how crops grew so well and abundantly in the middle of the desert.

So I set out to try and reproduce this water to drink myself and to witness firsthand if it had any special benefits.

This is when I began a serious review of Victor Schauberger's works I mentioned earlier on water modification. As well as his great works, I read some more recent research books on the topic of water, and I learned a fragment from everyone I read eventually coming up with this method that has been the only water not only I've consumed now for eight years but also my two cats have drunk as well.

Today, I call it by the name I also learned from my research of Giza Park—*rainbow water.*

This is the water I mentioned in my experiments that I felt I was getting about 30 percent of my energy calories from before I went ninety days with no food.

Enough historical talk, let's get to the recipe and instructions. *Rainbow water* is simple to make, a little labor intensive requiring about forty-eight hours' time from beginning using distilled water to finished product.

You will also need to fabricate or purchase at least two copper triskelion. I made my own using copper house wiring cut to 20.5 inches length and using needle nose pliers to bend. This is a very cheap method, and it's fun.

The 20.5-inch measurement I used is from the length of the sides of a cubit of measurement. This is a sacred number and is how the construction of the pyramids were measured.

Another comparison is during my bio-energetic research. It took me about two years to make a grid measurement of the human bio-energy field. When it was said and done, I calculated the human body's energy capacity in a simple measure is one cubit at 20.5 inches for each side. This means inches tall by 20.5 inches wide by 20.5 inches by 20.5 inches on the two sides.

There are a number of YouTube videos to choose from. Just YouTube triskelion construction.

Let me explain what these are as we go along. The triskelion is the oldest known symbol on earth, and it has been found carved in stones and megalithic structures all over the world by the created by the earliest humans.

I haven't been able to locate an opinion of any significance to the importance of the three spiral triskelion but there's been testing on what it does when fabricated out of copper.

Also on YouTube, you can watch a very good short video where a Kirlian camera that captures those frequencies shows the electric dynamic field produced by each spiral on the triskelion. Pretty beautiful and magnificent for me.

So I decided to use these to sit the distilled water on to create what is known as structuring the water. This is done because the triskelion are catching the earth's electromagnetic field and creating three torus fields or vortex energy flows. This not only slowly rotates the distilled water, it creates an electric field into the water equal to the earth's frequency.

This is a great thing because our human bodies are tuned to the exact same frequency as the earth. Our heart beats 7.3 MHZ, same as the earth's Schumann resonance frequency. In the end, this means that the distilled water changes its structure. It goes from a pure, harmful solvent to the human to a perfectly structure frequency that will allow this water to be easily absorbed deep into the mitochondria inside the cell.

A mitochondria is defined as an organelle found in large numbers in most cells, in which bio-chemical process of respiration and energy production occur.

This means that after sitting twenty-four hours on a triskelion, the distilled water changes and becomes able to go deeper into most cells of your body than anything you have ever consumed. That means rainbow water is also going to be a cleanse at first intake and therefore, needs to be taken in small increment. Same as sungazing—drink a glass today, two glasses tomorrow, next day three. You get the point. Soon you will be drinking it in your tea and coffee too. Imagine that first cup of Joe with an energy shot (lol).

(Warning! Consuming only distilled water will make you deathly ill. It is like a magnet to the minerals in your body; it sucks them out cleansing your cells.)

Another component of this first stage of processing I call the structuring, you need a small slab of granite to set the bottles on to structure. I prefer black granite based on research also. The ancients built all special structures and the most special statues out of black granite.

One, what does this mean? Well to me, it's this way: granite of varying qualities all contain a percentage of clear quartz crystal embedded in it. Inside the king's chamber of the Great Pyramid, the top beams of the ceiling are the heaviest stones in the pyramid and has the highest percentage of quartz crystal at 55 percent. And those stones are red granite, not black.

To explain further, you must understand how electricity works in a clear crystal. They are incredible rocks (lol).

Nikola Tesla said they were living creatures.

Today, all our computers rely on clear quartz crystals. Your cellphone needs crystals to operate, and all satellites in outer space would crash to earth without them at the helm.

This is how they work. It's called piezoelectric. What that means is a mechanical force that impacts the crystal causes a restructure of the crystal to the point it creates an electric spark. Let me explain it simply: you know that long lighter we use to light the grill, the fireplace, the candles, the one that has a trigger like a gun and you squeeze it and it clicks and amazingly fire appears at the end of that long tube? Basically that clicking sound is called a hammer and anvil like an old blacksmith beating metal to change its shape.

That hammer actually impacts a very small sliver of a clear quartz crystal glued at the bottom of that long tube. When the hammer strikes it, a spark is emitted from the crystal, and a wire has been glued to the back side of the crystal that carries that spark to the end of the barrel to ignite the butane gas pouring out.

Even though the clear quartz is not being hammered, it doesn't mean that the vibration of the earth doesn't charge these crystals, including the sun, because the greatest thing about the crystals is they never fail, and they are consistent in their voltage discharge. That means as many times as you can pull the trigger on that grill lighter, it will make a spark, and all of the sparks will have the identical current discharge for an indefinite period of time. Absolutely amazing!

Was Nikola Tesla correct? Are they living beings?

Okay, now we need containers for the water. I prefer half a gallon glass containers, like canning jars. I go through one gallon of my water a day on average, and that's a good number to figure. Two adults need two gallons.

I purchase my distilled water for convenience. One day, I want a distiller because for one person, you're hauling thirty gallons of water from grocery store to car to residence. For me, I live on a boat, and it's a three-quarter-mile walk from parking lot.

I must be crazy to go through this torture, but I believe it's worth it.

The next thing to do after filling the glass jars is to screw the lids on. Make sure they are plastic, not metal. Metal will create an interference to the energy fields we are manipulating.

Place the triskelion on the black granite that can hold two containers and set the filled containers atop of the triskelion. I typically let the containers sit here from eighteen to twenty-four hours. By this time, the water will be structured and energized to the feminine negative polarity.

Now comes the Himalayan pink salt super solution. This is the next step to creating an electrolyte to put into the water—same as a wet cell battery that starts your car engine.

I use a small glass jar that will hold approximately four ounces or a hundred fifty milliliters of liquid. Don't fill all the way up because you need to add one level tablespoon or fifteen milliliters of fine ground Himalayan pink salt to the distilled water. Place the lid back on the jar and shake furiously for a couple minutes to help dissolve the pink salt crystals.

I then set the super salt solution in a location where it is not disturbed so that the heavy materials can sink to the bottom. Himalayan pink salt contains eighty-four different minerals, and some of these are too large to dissolve. Let set over night. I usually take the lid off after shaking. That way, the next morning I don't reshake it to contaminate the solution with particles. We want it to be clear, not cloudy.

Okay, the next morning after the water is structured and the super salt solution has settled, I use an eye dropper and use one milliliter of the solution for each half a gallon container. What you have done now is created an electrolyte out of the structured distilled water.

Next is to find a sunny spot outside and set the containers to where the sun will shine on them for at least six to eight hours. One note is in the summertime of intense heat, do not allow the water to get hot. This degrades the energy capacity.

I never place my water in the refrigerator; I drink it at room temperature.

What we have done in this last step of placing in the sunlight is basically this. The water has been structured to a negative polarity. We added an electrolyte to it and then set it in the sunlight which is a positive masculine energy. The water then absorbs the solar plasma energy radiated from the sun like a magnet, literally creating a natural solar wet cell battery which contains real pure energy that can be used as calories—the same as if you were obtaining calories from food that you ate and had to digest and metabolize.

Thing about eating food as I stated earlier is no food ever enters into your blood stream. The calories all come from the chemical release of that energy as a frequency current. And it requires at least 50 percent of the calories you eat to digest, metabolize, and excrete as waste, so it is inefficient.

Therefore, the rainbow water requires very little processing and is perfectly structured for your cells.

Item List

2 Copper Triskelion 20.5 inches long
2 1/2 gallon glass jars for each person
1 Container of fine Himalayan pink salt
1 Small 4oz glass jar for super solution
1 Chunk of blank granite from countertop
1 Gallon of distilled water for each person
1 Eye dropper

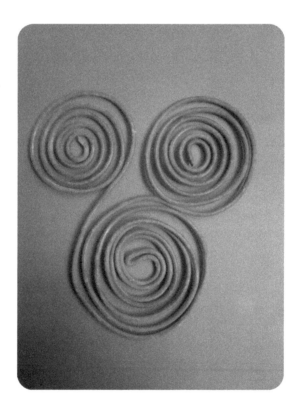

Chapter 18

Animals, Birds, Reptiles and Insects that Sungaze With New Insights on the Ancient Scarab Beetle

When addressing the topic of sungazing, I thought it appropriate to include some information about other creatures that inhabit the earth and owe their existence to the sun, sharing this common trait with man.

While this chapter will not be a complete list of the numerous species of creatures that I believe are active sungazers, I feel this representation offers sufficient evidence that suggests further scientific research should be directed into understanding this natural phenomena that has so many participants and goes across the thresholds of so many different species.

However, I can testify from my first-hand personal experiences of living afloat in a most special haven for the largest portion of the past twenty-seven years: a natural environment known as the Saltponds, an estuary of the Southern Chesapeake Bay in Virginia, USA. My direct experiences have been with birds, mostly the Great Blue Heron and the Yellow-crowned Night Heron when associated directly with sungazing.

My research over the years has produced some interesting evidence that relates to other species as well and some interesting symbolism that is associated with other cultures that dates back to the ancient Egyptians, that I cannot wait to share.

While this chapter was originally slated for publishing in this volume, it was almost lost over time as data collection became scattered about. I am very pleased to have discovered the missing data to include as a part of this publication.

I would like to begin by speaking of a very special bird I have had 100s and 100s of interactions with over the past seventeen years. For months of the year I have had several encounters with her a day, we have both become comfortable with each other and I can sometimes get as close to her as a few feet.

I named her Helen because of her beauty and my fondness for the ancient Greek epic poem attributed to Homer who penned some of the oldest works in Western Literature, including the great Odyssey. In his story and sequel to The Iliad, Homer told of the great battle of the famous Greek Hero Odysseus, king of Ithaca, and his ten year journey home after the fall of Troy. Which included the famous Trojan Horse, and a battle caused over revenge for a beautiful woman named Helen of Troy.

I feel this magnificent bird I named Helen recognizes her name, her intellect equal to her beauty. Helen is a Great Blue Heron and is the largest of the species I've seen here on the Chesapeake Bay.

Let me provide a little information about her species, her scientific name is Ardea Heodias and she is categorized as a wading bird. They are common near shores of open water and in wetlands across North America. Their average life span is fifteen years and one was documented that lived to be twenty-three years old; therefore Helen is ancient in her own right. I'll never forget that night, my first encounter with her, and she was an adult then, seventeen years ago.

I had just moved my motor yacht "Resurrected", a vessel I had salvaged and restored from a sinking accident from Windmill Point Marina off the Rappahannock River, to the Saltponds Marina, further south on the Chesapeake. I was enjoying a pleasant summer evening in my new digs. While I was laying on the foredeck of the vessel, Helen swooped out of the darkness, flying down across my body while screaming this horrible reptilian pterodactyl like sound. Between her landing call, which lasted seemingly, for an eternity and her huge size near five feet in length and with a wing-span over six

feet, I was startled to say the least by her grand entrance and introduction, as she landed just a few feet past my vessel, since I was
ported in the boat slip closest to the shore.

Ever since that night, our encounters became more and more
frequent and my fondness for her grew into adoration.

Looking back now, I can honestly say, I have never collected
as many photographic images of any other subject, which began in
35mm format transitioning to digital, as those of Helen. Because of
this, she became a topic of great interest. I've watched her habits and
studied her interactions with other birds and I feel I know her better
than anyone and I have become a bit of an expert on the species itself
because of her.

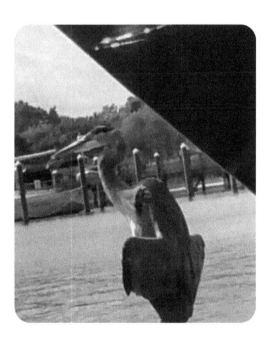

Over the years, one behavior she has that I began to take notice
of, is the habit of positioning herself into this odd posture. She always
stands on a hard surface such as the wooden docks or a piling at the
marina when she does it. I have never witnessed her once doing this
while standing in shallow water. She holds her body erect and facing the direction of the sun, and holds her wings from a downward

direction and fans them out to her sides looking like a satellite dish, similar as someone would use for a satellite antenna. She stays in this posture for lengthy periods never flinching, unless she is spooked by something, for an hour or longer periods.

It became obvious to me in 2013, when I first began my sungazing research, that this peculiar behavior Helen exhibited was definitely sungazing. It was during this period, when I noticed her doing this routine, I would quietly and indiscriminately, sneak as close to her as possible, without distracting or disturbing her, and I would sungaze with her.

Oh what a joy these encounters have always been! To have this type of experience is beyond description. As recently as a few days ago, I walked up on her sungazing and I stopped and shared a few minutes gaze time with her then, and it saddened me to realize my days at the Saltponds are short, as I am moving away soon.

Another bird I witnessed sungazing on occasion is another type of wading bird called a Yellow-crowned Night Heron, scientific name is the Nyctanassa violacea. This species is much smaller size and more shy than Helen's tribe. However, whenever they sungaze, the Night Heron follow a very similar method as the Great Blue Herons.

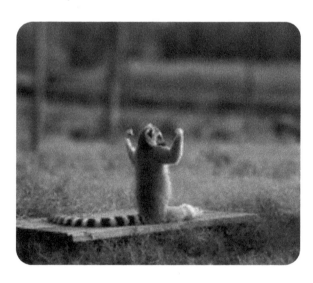

Ok, let's move on to an animal now that has a history of sun-gazing. That would be the adorable lemur. The lemur family has thirty-two different types of the primates in existence in the wild today and one of the favorites are found on the island of Madagascar. This particular Lemur are the endangered Ring-tailed Lemur. The Lemur catta is considered a large strepsirrhine primate and it is a diurnal species, which means it is active exclusively in daylight hours. Already, you can see a strong relationship with the sun. Sadly 95% of their population has disappeared since the year 2000.

The lemurs are known for gathering in groups, as many as thirty at a time and sunbathing sitting upright facing towards the sun. This posture is frequently described as a "sun-worshipping" posture and I like to compare it to the posture used by the ancient Jain Indians and Greeks. You have to wonder if these cultures didn't learn the method from these cute "sun-worshipping" primates?

Alright, while we always have considered reptiles as cold-blooded and logically would accept their natural close relationship with the sun to warm themselves up during the day. As a child and teenager, growing up in the mountains, it wasn't unusual to witness an occasional snake stretched out in the grass, soaking up the sunrays or going down to the river or numerous creeks and watching the turtles bask in the sun all day, seemingly dead, hardly ever moving.

There is one reptile that I discovered and is extremely curious to me, he looks like a small dragon and he has a peculiar relationship to the sun. Even his name gives us a clue to his addiction, as he is called the Sungazer Lizard. Also known as the Giant Girdled Lizard, this sun gazer goes by the scientific name Smaug Giganteus. He is a threatened species and is from the sub-Saharan Africa.

His lifestyle is much different than most lizards in his group that prefer to live amongst the rocks. The sungazers have a fancy for dirt and live in self excavated burrows, digging little tunnels over a foot deep and six feet in length in the silty soil of the grasslands in South Africa. They also live for an extended period of time, reaching twenty years of age, so they must be doing something right.

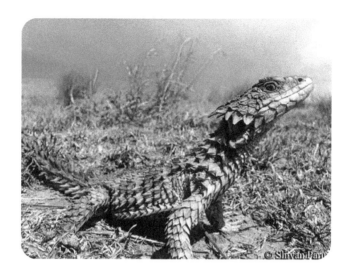

The species is well known as a sungazer, because of its thermo-regulatory behavior of elevating its anterior body parts by extending its fore limbs. It lays perched, from its burrow entrance as it looks at the sun. They have a well-known reputation amongst the locals, for spending most of the day in this sungazing posture sitting in the sunlight.

Alright, it is time to get ancient. Like ancient Egyptian. While we have data to suggest there are a number of insects that have a strong attachment to the sun, such as ants and bees, I want to focus on the beetle. Not just any beetle, but the stinkiest one, namely, the African Dung Beetle, of which there are about 2000 different species that exist in Africa today.

I chose this particular species because of the significant rela-tionship the Ancient Egyptians developed with the insect and also, there is a plethora of information to learn from that history. The African Dung Beetle was worshipped and held sacred by the Ancient Egyptians, that some claim built the pyramids. The pharaohs and their queens adorned themselves with exquisite jewelry of the beetles, many of the recovered art pieces show the beetle holding or looking at the sun.

What did this symbolism represent to the most powerful leaders of the time? Why would these powerful leaders want to be mum-

mified and entombed in ornate sarcophagus to spend eternity with
amulets, art and jewelry representing the dung beetle?

Let's explore the behavior of the dung beetle a little closer to see
if it makes any correlation.

To begin with, size for size, the dung beetle is the strongest
insect on the planet. Not only that, but they are the strongest animal
on the planet as well. When it comes to lifting weights, they are super
beetles, capable of lifting 1,141 times their weight. That's incredible.
To compare to a 150-pound human, he would have to be able to lift
171,150 pounds. Wow!

To relate just how extraordinary that beetle feat is, and to put
into perspective, an average school bus weighs 24,387 pounds. That
means that an average size man would have to be able to lift seven
school busses, to be equal in strength to that small insect, the scarab
beetle. Maybe this is one reason why the Egyptians were attracted to
the little guy. And when I say little guy, I use this description in the
masculine because the ancients believed all dung beetles were 100%
male species. Therefore, believing that male beetles had magical powers over the earth by being able to create life by injecting their life
force into the dung ball without the aid of a female.

Of course, scientist and researchers, have proven the Ancient
Egyptians were incorrect on this assumption, or that the assumption
had been more a political ploy to boost the superiority of the male
species at the time. After all, Ancient Egypt went through cycles of
masculine rule as well as feminine rule and many sacred monuments
were defaced or destroyed by the powers of authority who were in
power at the different cycles. This destructive behavior to monuments has been a historical legacy of humankind and is typical to
what's happening to monuments around the globe today.

One example the scarab beetle was used as a symbol to reflect
great strength was offered by the Pharaoh Amenhotep III, who ruled
from 1386 BCE to 1349 BCE. He used scarab beetles to reinforce
proclamations about his own personal greatness and the extent of his
power. There exist scarab beetles today from his period that boast his
great prowess at having personally killed 102 Lions.

Pharaoh Khepri, who reigned from the Dynastic Period, used the dung beetle to express his belief in resurrection, and he believed that death was not the end of life and rebirth was natural.

Later on, Yves Cambefort, a well-known French entomologist and dung beetle specialist, performed extensive research of scarab beetles. His findings led him to believe that many mummification rituals and methods can be compared to the idea of regeneration, via the dung beetles brood ball, creating a suitable environment for re-birth of the deceased pharaoh.

Cambefort even proposed that the interior chambers and tunnels of the burial tombs were similar to what the dung beetles construct themselves burrowing beneath the ground.

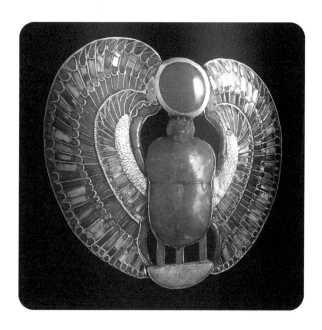

Myself, having attended the King Tutankhamun exhibition in December 2019 in London, there were numerous samples of mummified foods that were buried alongside of King Tut. This was a common ritual and provided the deceased a bounty of foods, so he would have sustenance once he awakened at the time of his re-birth.

It's also interesting that the life cycle of a dung beetle from fresh laid larva prior to emerging beetle takes 28 days, the same as the Moon cycle. The ancients felt the emergence of the dung beetle on the 29th day was the new regenerative cycle of the earth.

In Egyptian Astrology they used the scarab beetle to represent the sign of Cancer. It was much later that the Greeks and the Romans fashioned Cancer as the Crab that we accept today in the western astrology system.

Gathering some interesting scientific data, the species of dung beetle belong to the superfamily Scarabaeidae (Scarab Beetles) and they feed exclusively on feces. This group has 6,000 different species that are related. There is even one of these species that navigate and orient themselves using the Milky Way. Another species navigates by polarization patterns in moonlight. Again more amazing abilities.

Let's look at how long they have been on earth: dung beetles don't have bones so fossil records don't exist. However, dung balls have been found in fossils that were made by dung beetles and have been dated to over 30 million years ago. So dung beetles are some of the most ancient survivors on the planet.

Alright, let's segregate the dung beetles into the three categories scientist have established so we can better understand the Egyptians relationship and why they adored the insect: there is one group that is known as "dwellers", that live full time in the dung. There is a second group of "tunnellers" that dig below their pile of poop, so they can be close to their food source. Then the third group are the dung beetles that were indigenous to the North African region where the Giza Pyramids and other cities of ancient Egyptians thrived that were "rollers" of poop.

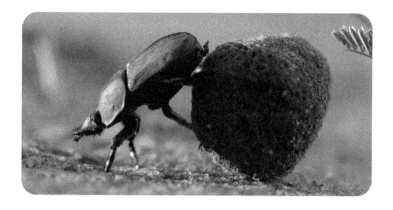

Yes, that's correct. These little guys will cling on to poop with their hind legs and roll the poop into rather large balls of poop. As a minority, only about ten percent of all dung beetles are called "rollers" and one of these species is the Scarabaeus Sacer. The exact same dung beetle that the Ancient Egyptians admired and used as the symbolic representative of numerous different ideals. They used the scarab beetle as a symbol of strength, immortality, resurrection, re-birth, transformation, and protection, all you can see expressed in their elaborate funerary art.

They felt that the life of the scarab beetle revolved around the dung balls: how the beetles consumed them for food, laid their eggs into the dung ball for birth, and fed their young represented the cycle of life and rebirth.

For me as a researcher I noticed in their beautiful art, the Egyptians often depicted the scarab beetle interacting directly with the sun. As we proceed, I have a theory to present that I feel offers collaboration to my beliefs about this common relationship with the sun that is absent from Egyptian history.

To understand the mechanics of propulsion the "rollers" use to transport the poop ball, and get the brood, to their home destination, is most bizarre. The scarab beetle, once he has completed fashioning and shaping the poop ball to his satisfaction, having rolled to the correct size, his next sequences of behavior has been studied and scrutinized extensively. The first thing the beetle does is he climbs atop of his poop ball and spins around in circles, orientating himself as to what direction he is to go to take his feast home.

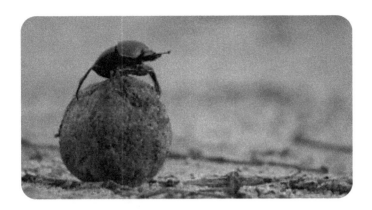

Once he has made his determination, he then climbs back down to ground level from the opposite side of the poop ball and that is the direction he needs to travel. He then places his head down towards the ground like he's doing a head stand and puts his rear legs up on the side of the poop ball and begins the relentless and awkward task of pushing against the poop ball, rolling it towards his destination while he is literally upside down and going backwards.

This is my question: How do the beetles know the correct direction to roll the poop ball to get it home when they cannot see where they are going?

Let's look at the latest research that was presented in a lecture on a Ted Talk by Marcus Byrne on December 13, 2012, titled, "The Dance of the Dung Beetle". His brief presentation, based on more than thirty years of field research in South Africa on dung beetles, proves without a doubt, the answer to my question. Marcus is a Professor in the School of Animal, Plant and Environmental Science at the University of the Witwatersrand, Johannesburg, Africa.

In 2019, Professor Byrne also co-authored and published a book based on his research with fellow Researcher Helen Lunn Ph.D. The text provides additional information that couldn't be presented in the short but informative twenty minute lecture, as is customary of Ted

Talk requirements. The printed version of their great experiments is titled, "Dance of the Dung Beetles" and is available in many formats.

Together, the two-scientist orchestrated many ingenious physical experiments where they created varying environments and mazes to test the Dung Beetles on their logic and natural process in three different categories. One was poop ball rolling, determining that the dung beetles practiced straight line navigation using celestial cues, namely the sun. Secondly, their experiments tested the beetles on their homing abilities, now learning they used path integration, which requires visual landmarks and is very much the same method of navigation used by ship captains known as "Dead Reckoning". Thirdly, what they classified as "The Dance", were the experiments they performed to determine how the dung beetles oriented themselves and used thermoregulation because of the significant temperatures generated from the mostly barren desert like conditions indigenous to Africa.

In their book, Byrne and Lunn reference the earlier research on dung beetles as reported by Horapollo, claiming that his research determined the Egyptians knew the posture the dung beetle positioned himself when rolling his poop ball. He said the dung beetles were always traveling westward because the beetle's eyes were focused on the sun in the east.

Another dung beetle researcher was mentioned as well, an Italian named Ulisse Aldrovandi, who solved the mystery of the dung beetle reproduction process and published his research in 1602. It took another 400 years, before an explanation about the influence the sun had on the orientation behavior of the dung beetle.

While I am not writing a thesis on dung beetles and will not detail their great experiments, I wanted to provide enough information to be able to offer an educated theory that collaborates my own research on the Giza Plateau. I literally became the obsessed, "mash potato" guy from the popular Spielberg movie, "Close Encounters of the Third Kind". I am sure Marcus Byrne and many other researchers understand this kind of "obsession" and have their own stories to tell.

My story began when my stepdaughter Rhayne, came home from school in the fourth grade, excited and carrying a library book explaining they had studied about the Great Pyramid that day in school. She couldn't wait to sit with me and go over what she had learned about the Pyramid and Egypt from her teacher.

Always encouraging the kids to read more and often reading to them myself, I was thrilled at her excitement and became all ears.

Let me tell you what I saw, and I was caught off guard and quite surprised. What I didn't realize at that moment, was how her enthusiasm was going to create an energy vision I witnessed, surrounding the Great Pyramid that I could physically see with my eyes. An energy system, that at the time I could obviously make out to look like wings. In reality the energy wasn't there. But for some odd reason, I could see it. I even asked her, and she denied seeing the energy field. The energy flowed around the outside structure of the Great Pyramid, and at that moment, my life changed direction. I suddenly became obsessed with Egypt. So obsessed, that several years later Rhayne's mom divorced me because she said, "she was tired of living in fucking Egypt".

First, I need to set the scene. At that time, I had absolutely no interest in Egypt or pyramids, and I wasn't familiar with scarab beetles or that culture's history. Yes, years earlier I had seen a documentary about the Great Pyramid and the Sphinx.

My interest of research was bio-energetics and I had been sourcing many volumes on that topic. I had discovered the bio-energy research works of Christopher Hills, who had created a New Age University in California in the '70s, known as the "University of the Trees." I had picked up his book at a recent visit to Edgar Casey's ARE, and his great library in Virginia Beach, Virginia.

I learned of the "University of the Trees" and observed the agenda of this this faculty: the subjects taught were much different than the typical university in the U.S. It did include some standard classes on art, literature, environmental studies, alternative energy systems, health and yoga. But it also offered courses in transpersonal awareness, history of neurology of consciousness, mysticism, radiational physics, including radiesthesia, dowsing and pyramid research.

Hills work on the Giza pyramids was all related to bio-energies inside the Great Pyramid and I had read his methods and discoveries.

It was interesting the synchronistic timing of events. I had been discussing the Great Pyramid with the family and the school system only teaches about the Giza Plateau pyramids just one day total during the twelve year education system locally. So, Rhayne was excited because she had just learned about the Great Pyramid at home and after listening to her teacher's lecture, became even more excited and interested in pyramids. She went to the school library that day and checked out a book about the pyramids to bring home and share with me.

However, as I was energetically moved by her excitement as she repeated what her teacher had said that day, my eyes became fixed on an image of the Great Pyramid that I couldn't ignore and became distracted.

I saw a multicolored energy field that surrounded the exterior of the Great Pyramid that rose up above it and my first thought was that they reminded me of wings, like from a colorful butterfly. The energies created an arc-like configuration that was shaped similar to the Ankh, the wings were attached to the earth on both sides of the stone constructed structure.

Honestly, it was sometime later that I determined the wing-like energy field was that of the scarab beetle.

As I began researching the scarab beetle and recognizing the addition of the sun in most of the symbology, it finally became clear and made sense, and I drew the image presented here. I've learned it is not unusual for me that I draw the sketches I see in my mind first and later understand the meanings. That's just the way it is with me.

As my research matured, fueled by my obsessions, I determined how all of the systems operated at the Giza Plateau and integrated with one another. I am convinced my 100s of drawings and 1000s of pages of written research is the most complete systems analogy of the Giza Plateau since they were constructed. This included not just the structures constructed on the land that is visible, but I also took into account all of the systems that had been constructed below the ground as well.

This book your reading now would have never been written if that day had not occurred when Rhayne showed me the Great

Pyramid images. The recipe for my rainbow water at the end of this text was developed from my discoveries about the Great Pyramid and how the systems integrate with each other on the Giza Plateau.

Looking back now, I want to explain exactly how following a decade's amount of research on the Giza Plateau has made me believe certain details about the symbolic representation of the scarab beetle. I am convinced without a doubt that my concepts reflect well beyond the scope of knowledge that the Ancient Egyptians had at the time.

Now, it is easy to understand why they revered the scarab beetle and they had many reasons, based on the information I have presented for discussion.

In summation, I feel that my discoveries reinforce, with substantial collaborative evidence, and support the views, unequivocally, the existing theories similar to the famed archeologist John Anthony West and geologist Robert Schoch. I agree that the Sphinx and most likely the pyramids themselves are much older than what is currently accepted as when the Giza Plateau Systems were constructed.

My attempt to understand the established time frames that is sold to the general public by the Egyptian Historical Society which suggest for example that the Pharaoh Kufu constructed the Great Pyramid as fact. Or the claims by Egyptologist that the second larger pyramid named Kafrae and the smaller Menkaure were also the builders has absolutely no physical evidence and I consider those as opinions and are designed to attract tourist dollars, not provide accurate historical data.

I am convinced that Kufu during his reign hadn't a clue as to why the pyramids were built or how they operated. I see him standing in front of the Great Pyramid screaming to the heavens, "*Why?*"

I can only assume the Ancient Egyptians most likely would not have had the knowledge to be able to associate the scarab beetle in relation to how the pyramids functioned. It seems if they understood they would have left explanations as to how and why, which they did not.

I am convinced the scarab beetle was also a symbol that related to how the pyramids themselves on the Giza Plateau interfaced with the sun.

My visions led me, as a systems guy, to understand the Great Pyramids systems, which once learned, opened my eyes to examine the other components and determine that I was dealing with a huge and powerful industrial facility. An industrial park that was constructed with a specific purpose and was engineered and designed by those who understood energies much better than we do today.

With this being stated, I believe that the entire Giza Plateau, on and below the ground, and some of the surrounding areas, were all systems of operations for a magnificent industrial park, I coined as "Giza Park".

I used the "Emerald Tablets" expressed by Hermes Trismegistus as my "blueprints" to follow as guides on determining the function of many of the systems. One for example, "As Above, So Below" which describes all the systems, even when in operation.

The Giza Plateau Industrial Park, so well-constructed that the builders used all indigenous natural components that existed near-by and integrated them together. Using an advanced understanding of quantum entanglement, these methods can only be classified as most genius. The designers created a massive site, on a site located in the perfect energy location, to create influence on weather, climate, and land mass disassociation. On one cycle it operated for 5,300 years, creating sufficient energy in the heat medium to turbo charge the earth's incidental solar radiation, raising the high temperatures associated with deserts significantly enough to melt the last Ice Age in a remarkable short period of time.

I used the results of the International Scientist collaborative efforts, borrowing the same scientific mathematical calculations they used, to figure the "Incidental Solar Radiation" of the African Desert. I utilized my discoveries with the data the science investigators created on determining the amount of energy on earth available to melt the 2,000 mile-thick ice sheet that blanketed a large portion of the Northern Hemisphere in a shortened time frame of about 5,000 years.

My determination was that Giza Park was a major system that significantly influenced the acceleration of melting the Ice Age in a period at least 100,000 years sooner than could have been accomplished based on the natural energies available upon the earth at that time. The scientific mystery since the '70s that have baffled scientist to the degree that they gave up on trying to solve what is known as the "Energy Paradox".

Without any further explanations of the "Energy Paradox" theories which will be explained in future text to follow this one, I want to return to the scarab beetle now that I've explained the great significance this symbology represents to me based on my research and discoveries related to the Giza Plateau.

I also have to admit, without any physical evidence to present at this time, that it is very possible that the Giza System may very well be at least 13,000 years older and the system may have been operated multiple times over the centuries. Functional, at times when they were necessary, to create changes to the environment on earth to facilitate human survival, expansion and abundance.

As I stated earlier, I was steered in this regard by Hermes' "Emerald Tablets" and by predictions made by the psychic Edgar Casey. "As Above, So Below" was my "Boiler Plate" that I used as a guide, and I stayed true to that mantra and everything just dropped into place. It was during that time that I made the association of the Giza systems I named Giza Park, determining it was an industrial park and was a very hazardous environment when the facility was in operation mode.

I had determined the relationship between the sun and Sirius and understood the synchronicity of the "Helical Sunrise".

I also figured out how all the systems functioned and integrated with each other and determined that Nikola Tesla had understood the pyramids the same as me. He designed not only the "Waldenclyffe Tower" on Long Island, New York, but also the "HAARP" facility in Alaska, realizing both of these projects were designed to interact energetically with the earth's ionosphere when making a direct connection to the sun.

The ionosphere itself is fueled by solar radiation, it is an active ocean of superheated plasma that contains a high concentration of ions and free electrons. It begins at about thirty miles above the earth and is about 600 miles thick. The temperature of the ionosphere has a variable temperature range depending on the influence of the sun, via night to day. The temperature at night can be -100 degrees Fahrenheit to 440 degrees Fahrenheit during the daytime.

Now we can see the direct influence the sun has on the ionosphere, making the ionosphere diurnal in its hottest temperature and most powerful during the daytime; exactly the same influence on the diurnal schedule of the dung beetle.

Also, in my discoveries I determined that the Giza Park industrial park was also a diurnal operating system and I made the connection with collaborative information I gathered about this sacred scarab beetle.

Therefore, I am convinced that one symbolic representation of the dung beetle had been unrecognized by what we consider the Ancient Egyptians as well. This only collaborates that Giza Park is older than their civilization and adds more evidence that proves they inherited the pyramids from an earlier, unknown advanced civilization. Therefore, since they did not design or build the systems, they had no understanding of most of the symbolism they claimed as their own and this explains why that information has been lost today.

If my theories are correct about the systems operation and function of Giza Park, we have to recognize the distinct possibility that the pyramids themselves are significantly influenced by the sun to be diurnal operating systems only functional during the day.

In closing, I want to list the topics discussed in the later part of this chapter with the diurnal relationships with the sun. Beginning with the scarab beetle, the ionosphere, the pyramids, Giza Park and of course the sun.

To identify all these relationships to be connected directly to the sun is a great way to end this volume.

To be continued...

Bibliography

Aivanhov, Omraam Mikhael. *Life Force.* France: Prosveta S.A., 2004.
———. *Man's Subtle Bodies and Centers.* France: Prosveta S.A., 2009.
———. *Spiritual Alchemy.* France: Prosveta S.A., 2008.
———. *The Second Birth: Love Wisdom Truth.* France: Prosveta S.A., 2009.
———. *The Splendour of Tiphareth, The Yoga of the Sun.* France: Prosveta S.A., 2001.
———. *The True Meaning of Christ's Teaching.* France: Prosveta S.A., 20011.
———. *Toward a Solar Civilization.* France: Prosveta S.A., 2008.
Andres, Frank. *Nikola Tesla-Ocean of Eyes.* USA: Frank W. Andes, 2013.
Austin-Sparks, T. *Rivers of Living Water.* USA: Witness and Testimony, 1957.
Bartholomew, Alick. *Hidden Nature.* USA: Floris Books, 2003.
Budge, E.A. Wallis *Egyptian Book of the Dead.* United Kingdom: Penguin Group, 2008.
Byrne, Marcus and Lunn, Helen. *Dance of the Dung Beetles/Their Role in our Changing World*, South Africa, Wits University Press, 2019
Case, Mary J. *Qi Gong Movements for Hands and Wrist.* USA: Mary J. Case, 2013.
Charak, K.S. *Surya the Sun God.* United Kingdom: Aadyaa Books, 2010.
Culling, Louis T., and Carl Llewellyn Weschcke. *The Complete Magic Curriculum of the Secret Order G.B.G.* USA: Llewellyn Publications, 2013.
Dauno, Beinsa. Food and Water: Messages from Heaven.

Doreal, M. *The Emerald Tablets of Thoth the Atlantean*. USA: Bear and Company, 1998.

Dunn, Christopher. *The Giza Power Plant: Technologies of Ancient Egypt*. USA: Bear and Company, 1998.

Dwinell, LAC, Mason Howe. *The Earth was Flat*. USA: Xlibris US, 2005.

Emoto, Masaru. *The Hidden Messages in Water*. USA: Atria Books, 2011.

Farber, Phillip H. *Brain Magic*. USA: Llewellyn Publications, 2011.

Finklea, Bob. *Sun Gazing, How Millions of Ancient Peoples used the Sun to Heal Themselves and Perform Miracles*. USA: Web Media Central, 2014.

Gienger, Michael, and Joachim Goebel. *Gem Water*. United Kingdom: Earth Dancer GMBH, 2008.

Gray, Elisha. *Electricity and Magnetism*. USA: Public Domain/Amazon, 2011.

Hall, Manly. *Secret Teachings of All Ages*. Germany: Jazzybee-Verlag Jurgen Beck, 1928.

Hall, Manly. *The Energy Fields of the Human Body*. USA: Barabbas Publishers, 2016.

Hills, Christopher, *Supersensonics: The Spiritual Physics of all Vibrations from Zero to Infinity (The Supersensitive Life of Man)*, USA, University of the Trees Press, 1978.

Hoffman, Daniella Rama. *The Tablets of Light: The Teachings of Thoth on Unity Consciousness*. Canada: Bear and Company/Simon and Schuster, 2017.

Holick, Michael F. *The UV Advantage*. USA: Bricktower Press, 2003.

Holman, Andy. *Breathing Secrets*. USA: Andy Holman Published, 2013.

Jasmuheen. *Four Body Fitness: Biofields and Bliss*. Australia: Self Empowerment Academy, 2001.

———. *The Food of the Gods*. Australia: Self Empowerment Academy, 2003.

———. *Pranic Nourishment-Living on Light*. Australia: Self Empowerment Academy, 1996.

Jhon, Mu Shik. *The Water Puzzle and the Hexagonal Key.* Korea: Uplifting Press, 2004.

Jones, Robert, Dr. MD, PHD, DDS, ODD and Porup Jim. *Food-Free at Last: How I Learned to Eat Air.* USA: American Journal of Atmospheric Consumption, 2012.

Le Page, Joseph and Lilian. *Mudras: For Healing and Transformation.* USA: tegrative Yoga Therapy, 2013.

LeCram, Irene. *The Sun Gazer.* USA: Self published LeCram, 2012.

Liberman, Jacob. *Light: Medicine of the Future.* USA: Bear and Company, 1990.

————. *Take Off Your Glasses and See.* USA: Three Rivers Press, 1995.

Lingane, Mark. Tesla (Evolution Book 1). USA: Insync Books, 2013.

Manek, Hira Ratan "HRM." *Living on Sunlight, The Art and Science of Sun Gazing.* Edited by Vina Parmar, MBA. USA: as Living on Sunlight Publishing, 2004.

McCloud, Ace. *Eye Sight and Vision Cure.* USA: Self Published Ace McCloud, 2013.

Murdock, D.M. *Jesus as the Sun.* USA: Stellar House Publishing, 2011.

Pangmanand, MJ, and Melanie Evans. *Dancing With Water: The New Science of Water.* USA: Self Published MJ Pangmanand and Melanie Evans, 2011.

Pollack, Gerald H. *The Fourth Phase of Water.* USA: Ebner and Sons Publishers, 2013.

Rasbold, Eric and Katrina. *Energy Magic.* USA: Rasbold Ink, 2014.

Reich, Wilhelm. *Orgonomy.* USA: Farrar, Straus and Guroud, 2013.

Rice, James Michael. *For Those that Worship the Sun.* USA: Self Published James Michael Rice, 2013.

Salvitti, Tony. *Longevity.* USA: Self Published Anthony Salvitti, 2012.

Schauberger, Viktor. *Nature as Teacher.* United Kingdom: Gill Macmillian Books, Translation by Callum Coats, 1968.

————. *The Water Wizard.* United Kingdom: Gill Books, 1999.

Seifer, Marc J. *Wizard, The Life and Times of Nikola Tesla: Biography of a Genius.* USA: Ciadel Press, Kensington Publishing Corp., 1968.

Shealy, C. Norman. *Energy Medicine.* USA: 4th Dimension Press, 2011.

Smith, Jane Ma'ati. *The Emerald Tablet of Heremes and the Kybalion.* USA: Created Space, Independent Publishing Platform, 2008.

Steiner, Rudolf. *Egyptian Myths and Mysteries.* USA: Globel Grey, 2013.

Stiene, Bronwen and Frans. *The Reiki Sourcebook.* USA: John Hunt Publishing, 2010.

Stith, Casper. *The Day Free Energy Died: Nikola Tesla's Nightmare.* USA: Self Published Casper Stith, 2015.

Stockl, Michael Thomas. *Life From Light: Is it Possible to Live Without Food?* Germany: Clairview, 2012.

Taylor, Jill Bolte. *My Stroke of Insight.* USA: Penguin Group, 2006.

Tennant, Jerry L. *Healing is Voltage: The Handbook.* USA: Self Published Jerry Tennant, 2013.

Tesla, Nikola. *The Illustrated Tesla.* USA: Sublime Books, 2013.

———. *Imagination and the Man that Invented the 20th Century.* USA: Self Published Sean Patrick, 2020.

———. *My Inventions, Autobiography.* USA: Start Publishing LLC, 2012.

———. *Nikola Tesla: The Controversial Story and Secrets of the Famous Inventor of Electricity.* USA: Self Published Timothy Bauer, 2013.

———. *On Light and Other High Frequencies.* USA: Start Publishing LLC, 2012.

———. *Talking with Planets.* USA: Paphos Publishing, 2015.

———. *The Lost Journals of Nikola Tesla.* USA: Global Communications, 2011.

———. *The Problem of Increasing Human Energy, With Special Influences to Harnessing of Sun's Energy.* USA: Public Domain Nikola Tesla, 1900.

———. *The Strange Life of Nikola Tesla.* USA: Dragan Nikolic Aristeus Books, 2012.

———. *Very Truly Yours, Nikola Tesla.* USA: Wilder Publications, 2014.

———. Quotations. USA: Self Published Urszula Miller, 2013.

Tu Tai Chi Club. *Qi Gong 10 Postures*. United Kingdom: Tai Chi Club, 2013.

Yogananda, Paramahansa. *Autobiography of a Yogi*. China: Crystal Clarity Publishers, 1946 reprint 2015.

———. *The Bhugavad Gita*. USA: Self-Realization Fellowship, 2018.

Waits, DC. *Tesla's Strange Experiments: Time Traveler Death Ray Spaceships*. USA: Self Published DC Waits, 2014.

Warner, Lisa. *The Simplicity of Self-Healing*. USA: Self Published Lisa Warner, 2013.

About the Author

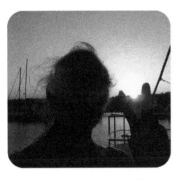

Captain Leo Walton grew up in the mountains of Virginia, a youth spent camping and doing sports such as water skiing and track. Finishing his early schooling, he relocated to the East Coast to further his education and train as a nuclear apprentice helping to construct and refuel nuclear navy vessels. Learning how shipboard systems functioned with hands-on experience from the Aircraft Carriers Enterprise, Nimitz, Vincent, the Frigates California, South Carolina, Virginia to the Los Angeles Class Submarines.

Looking for a career change, Captain Leo became a professional firefighter performing emergency services for two different communities.

Acting on an opportunity some years later, Captain Leo re-entered into the manufacturing and production environment where he was responsible for plant support systems, emergency services, and R&D.

It was during this decade Captain Leo had two US patents approved creating the first ergonomic designed runners' water bottles, which were marketed around the globe.

Heeding to new opportunities, Captain Leo once again changed careers which led him to becoming responsible for the set-up of two new companies in his local community. The later one of his responsibilities was as project manager/engineer to remove, re-engineer, and reinstall the fire suppression pump which supplied the sprinkler systems and fire hoses used by the firefighters to attempt to contain the flames inside the tall structures. This pump was responsible for allowing fifty thousand people to flee and escape to safety from the Twin Towers buildings on 9/11 before they came crashing down.

It was an extraordinary sequence of events to follow from the destruction of Twin Towers in America. Captain Leo became a Plank founding member of Homeland Security due to his ownership of a USCG merchant marine captain's license.

Captain Leo's love of the water, having sailed over twenty-five thousand nautical miles and living afloat for twenty-six years, always had high ambitions and wanted one day to own a company of his creation. So he diligently and carefully structured a successful marine forensics investigation company. For fifteen years, Captain Leo performed over two thousand five hundred forensics investigations, representing nineteen insurance companies and consulting on seven hurricane catastrophe teams.

After an accidental electrocution while working aboard his own vessel in 2007, Captain Leo's successful life changed dramatically. His "grand illumination," as he calls it, ended his career, marriage, and quality of life.

Over time, Captain Leo was able to incorporate all his life experiences and curiosity, using his investigative skills and systems understanding to investigate and research many ancient mysteries, creating new theories and perspectives never presented before.

The Captain has numerous projects to produce additional titles to share from the purpose and systems function of the Giza Pyramids, the Energy Paradox related to the termination of the Ice Age, the races of giants and elongated skull civilizations, the Nazca Lines, earth energy grids, the Bermuda Triangle to the mystery of why the electromagnetic north field is moving thirty-four miles west every year.

This volume is the first of thirteen manuscripts with one being turned into a movie adaptation.

CPSIA information can be obtained
at www.ICGtesting.com
Printed in the USA
LVHW072055150722
723643LV00008B/48